# HEART ATTACKS, HYPERTENSION, AND HEART DRUGS

# HEART ATTACKS, HYPERTENSION, AND HEART DRUGS

M. Gabriel Khan, M.D.
M.B., B.Ch., M.D. (Queen's Belfast),
M.R.C.P. (London), F.R.C.P. (C), F.A.C.P.
Consultant Cardiologist, Physician in Charge,
Clinical Teaching Unit, Ottawa General Hospital;
Associate Professor of Medicine,
University of Ottawa,
Ottawa, Canada

**SEAL BOOKS**
McClelland and Stewart-Bantam Limited
Toronto

HEART ATTACKS, HYPERTENSION, AND HEART DRUGS
*A Seal Book / June 1986*

**Canadian Cataloguing in Publication Data**

Khan, M. Gabriel.
    Heart attacks, hypertension and heart drugs

(Canadian medical library)
Bibliography: p.

1. Coronary heart disease.    2. Coronary heart
disease—Prevention.    3. Hypertension.
4. Heart—Effect of drugs on.    I. Title.    II. Series.

RC685.C6K48    1986        616.1'23        C86-093501-9
ISBN 0-770-42125-3

PRINTED IN CANADA

COVER PRINTED IN U.S.A.

CW        0  9  8  7  6  5  4  3  2  1

Dedicated to
the glory of God
—the truth the light and the way.
Perhaps praise should be silent;
should I not utter it when I can.

# NOTICE

---

The author and the publisher cannot be held responsible for damages incurred by patients in using the information given in this book, be it related to nondrug or drug treatment. Patients are strongly advised to follow the directives of their doctor at all times. The information given in this book is to be used only along with the advice of your doctor.

The Author and Publisher

# CONTENTS

# ACKNOWLEDGEMENTS

Thanks must go to Maureen Ivan, who assisted with editing the manuscript; to Emile Purgina, graphic artist, University of Ottawa School of Medicine; to Debbie Willems Nyenkamp for her word processing skills and to all my friends and patients who read parts of the manuscript and offered suggestions. The contributions of my daughter Christine, Jim Tayler and Tim Kehoe are greatly appreciated; as well I wish to thank my wife and children for their help and support.

# PREFACE

A heart attack is caused by the narrowing and finally the block-age of a coronary artery (coronary heart disease). Each year more than a million Americans experience a heart attack. About a half million of these die within one hour of the onset of symptoms (sudden cardiac death). About a half million survive to reach the hospital. The death rate in hospitals is about 15 percent. About 425,000 patients survive to leave hospitals, and approxi-mately 10 percent (42,000) of these die within the next year. It has been shown that 33 percent of these deaths can be pre-vented by beta-blocking drugs (beta-blockers).[1] Therefore, about 14,000 lives can be saved in the United States annually, and as many nonfatal heart attacks can be prevented. Coronary heart disease costs the United States more than $60 billion a year in direct health care costs, lost productivity, and wages.

The public needs to be educated and motivated to reduce their risk of heart attack. Officially, high blood pressure, high blood cholesterol, and smoking are major culprits termed "risk factors." Intensive research during the 1980s has resulted in new information and changes in nondrug and drug treatment recommendations. Therefore, in Part I, I have devoted a chap-ter to each risk factor, and I provide answers to questions such as, "Is cholesterol important again?" and "Can one aspirin taken daily prevent heart attacks?" Stress may be as important as the three major risk factors but it is not easy to validate scientifi-cally the role of stress. However, in the chapter on stress I have outlined recent experiments that shed light on stress and the heart.

A blood clot in the coronary artery (coronary thrombosis) causes the heart attack in the majority of patients. Can we prevent the clot from forming? There is little or no information on this subject in available books directed at the public. Books on prevention of heart attacks emphasize only the risk factors. Based on the results of recent research, new ideas will be outlined to help you to understand how you can prevent blood clot formation and heart attack.

I have not included diet plans and recipes because they are often not applicable to the individual. Such diets are difficult to follow for a lifetime. Therefore, I have given you clear instructions so that you can arrange for yourself what I term "A Sensible Heart Diet." It involves advice derived from the American Heart Association's Prudent Heart Diet and more recent information that relates to the possible prevention of blood clots by special foods.

Part I also gives scientific as well as common sense advice on exercise and stress with the hope that you will learn to live and enjoy a happier, relaxed, and more peaceful life.

Part II discusses the treatment doctors use for a heart attack as well as what you must do to achieve better and quicker recovery. I must emphasize that the "new drug treatment" to dissolve clots in the coronary artery has a chance of success only if it is given within four hours of onset of symptoms. After about four hours, the area of affected heart muscle dies and function to this area cannot be restored. I have clearly outlined the various symptoms and signs of a heart attack so that the public can learn to recognize them and thus go quickly to an appropriate hospital to receive this new treatment. Perhaps in the 1990s such treatment may be available in the home.

Given that angina (recurrent chest pain) is a very common heart condition, I have detailed relevant drug information that I feel you are entitled to know. At times I state why one drug is superior and another useless, bearing in mind the high cost of drugs.

Part III describes hypertension in detail. This condition, which affects about 60 million North Americans and contributes to about a million deaths from heart attack and a half million strokes annually, merits detailed discussion. Therefore, I have devoted a chapter to this important preventable and curable condition. I have given information on nondrug management as well as advice on how the doctor and the individual should go about selecting the best drug from the many antihypertensive drugs now available.

This book is based on my twenty years of experience

managing patients with heart disease and hypertension. However, I must emphasize that the suggested treatment schedules are not simply my own but are derived from a thorough review of the world literature on nondrug and drug management of cardiac conditions.

Only the generic names of drugs are given in the text; the reader will find the pharmaceutical trade names in Appendix A. You should use the information in this book only along with the advice of your doctor.

# HOW TO PREVENT HEART ATTACKS

# CHAPTER 1

# DEFINITIONS AND CAUSES

The patient with a heart attack is suddenly stricken by pain in the center of the chest. The pain is often unbearable but can be a pressure-like discomfort associated with difficult breathing, profuse sweating, and a strange frightened feeling. The cause of a heart attack in the majority of cases is a blockage of a coronary artery that feeds the heart muscle with blood containing oxygen, glucose, sodium, potassium, calcium, and other nutrients. In more than 90 percent of patients, the blockage has been shown conclusively to be due to a blood clot.[2] The blood clot is often present on the surface of a partially obstructing plaque of atheroma (atherosclerosis) that shows fissuring (rupture or ulceration). The blocked artery cuts off blood to a segment of heart muscle (myocardium), the cells of which die because they are deprived of the nutrients in the blood. This death of heart muscle cells is termed a myocardial infarction (Figure 1-1). After a few months this area of dead muscle forms a well-healed scar. The size of the myocardial infarction depends on the coronary artery affected, i.e., a main vessel or a branch artery, and what part of the heart muscle it supplies. A heart attack is synonymous with the term "myocardial infarction" and, for practical purposes, with "coronary thrombosis."

In many patients who die suddenly, within one hour of the onset of symptoms, their attack is triggered by an electrical disturbance termed ventricular fibrillation, during which the heart "quivers" and does not contract. Previous studies indicated that more than half of these patients had no evidence of a blood clot in the coronary artery, but a recent study indicates

3

# Fig. 1-1 Coronary Heart (Artery) Disease

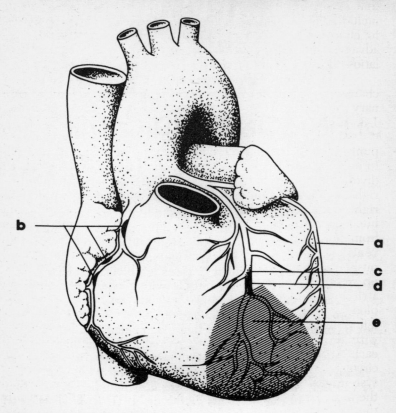

a) **Normal coronary artery**
b) **Obstruction of a coronary artery by atherosclerosis causing less blood to reach the heart muscle, producing chest pain, called angina.**
c) **Blood clot**
d) **Complete obstruction of a coronary artery by atherosclerosis and blood clot (coronary thrombosis), causing (e)**
e) **Damage and death of heart muscle cells, ie., a heart attack (myocardial infarction).**

that a clot (coronary thrombosis) is present in most patients, including those who die suddenly.[3] Intensive research is needed to clarify this very important area and to investigate recent advances that shed light on the prevention of ventricular fibrillation through drug therapy in patients at high risk.

At this point, I must provide you with information on the characteristic action of various parts of the heart, on the coronary arteries, and on atheroma, or atherosclerosis (Figures 1-2, 1-3, 1-4).

The human heart is a muscular pump. Its function is to pump blood containing oxygen, glucose, protein, fat, and salts to every organ, tissue, and living cell of the body. The heart is divided into four chambers. The upper chambers are called the right and left atrium, and the lower chambers are called the right and left ventricle. Blood from all parts of the body drains into veins that empty into the right atrium. The blood passes from the right atrium through a valve and reaches the right ventricle. During contraction of the right ventricle, blood is pushed into the lungs, where it gives off carbon dioxide, takes up oxygen, and returns via the pulmonary veins to the left atrium (Figure 1-2). During relaxation of the left ventricle, the blood passes from the left atrium through a valve to reach the left ventricle. When the left ventricle contracts, simultaneously with the right, about 70 milliliters of blood are ejected with each heartbeat through the aortic valve into the aorta and circulated through the branches of the aorta that form the arterial system and supply blood to organs and tissues of the body. If the heart beats 70 times per minute, it produces an output from the heart of approximately 5 liters of blood per minute; this is called the cardiac output. Each 70 milliliters of blood is propelled through approximately 100,000 kilometers of blood vessels. The heart beats about 2.5 billion times during an average life span, pumping more than 227 million liters of blood. Fortunately, the heart muscle is one of the strongest in the body. It can maintain efficient pumping and life for more than a hundred years provided that the coronary arteries that feed the muscle with blood do not become blocked by hardened plaques or a blood clot.

*The coronary arteries* run along the outer surface of the heart (Figure 1-3). There are two main coronary arteries, left and right, which originate at the root of the aorta as it leaves

# Figure 1-2. Structure of the Heart

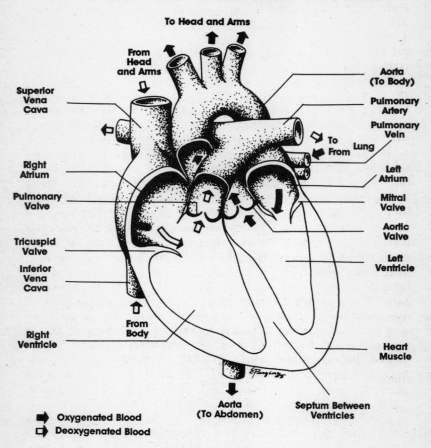

the heart. The left main coronary artery is very short, 0.1 to 4 centimeters, and divides almost immediately into two branches. The first branch called the anterior descending artery, runs down the front or anterior surface of the heart, near the under-surface of the left margin of the breastbone. It supplies blood to a major portion of the left ventricle. The second branch, called the circumflex artery, circles around and feeds the back of the heart. The right coronary artery leaves the aorta, veers sharply left, then is directed toward the breastbone and curves down-ward to run along the border of the right ventricle. The right coronary artery supplies branches to the electrical system, which involves special cells that cause the heart to beat (the sinus node pacemaker), and to the conducting bridge for electrical transmission between the atrium and ventricle (atrio-ventricular node). The branches subdivide several times and perforate the heart muscle at different points to bring nutrients to the mus-cle. These arteries have nothing to do with the blood flow inside the heart, which is pumped around the body. In addi-tion, their internal diameter is only about the size of a soda straw. Arteries are tubes which carry blood; the channel within a tube is the lumen.

You can consider the heart as being supplied by four arteries, the left main coronary artery, the left anterior de-scending, the circumflex, and the right coronary arteries. It is easy to visualize blockage of the left main coronary artery as the most dangerous, as it would block off two major arteries. Fortu-nately, this occurrence is rare. Most heart attacks are due to blocks in the right coronary artery, the anterior descending, and less commonly, the circumflex, or smaller branches of these three arteries.

Blockage of the coronary artery by atherosclerosis is ex-tremely common and more than 50 percent of North American males over age thirty-five and females over age fifty have signif-icant plaques of atheroma partially obstructing one or more coronary arteries. These partially obstructing plaques of ather-oma jut into the lumen of the artery and disturb the free flow of blood to the heart muscle. The plaques do not usually cause symptoms, but in some individuals, chest pain (angina) occurs on exertion because the partially obstructed artery cannot sup-ply enough blood and oxygen during exertion. The pain of

## Figure 1-3.  Coronary Arteries

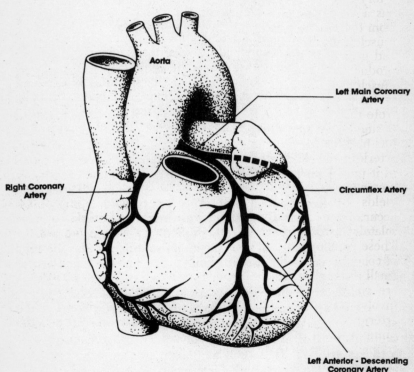

angina disappears quickly if the individual stops the precipitating activity.

~ *Atherosclerosis* is a form of arteriosclerosis. The latter denotes a hardening of arteries due to all causes, including calcification, loss of elasticity, atheroma, and others. The word "atheroma" is derived from the Greek stem "athera," meaning porridge or gruel. When a plaque of atheroma is cut, one can see a gelatinous, thick, porridge-like material, which contains cholesterol and other fatty material. The plaque of atheroma involves the inner lining (intima) and the middle wall of the artery (Figure 1-4). Apart from a rich fat content, the plaque has a preponderance of smooth muscle cells that are derived from the middle part of the arterial wall (media). These smooth muscle cells are believed to be very important in the formation and growth of the plaque. Substances such as cholesterol and products released from blood platelets stimulate the smooth muscle cells to proliferate, thus enlarging the plaque.

A cross section of a coronary artery is shown in Figure 1-4. Note that the inner wall of the artery in contact with the blood is smooth. When atherosclerosis occurs, a plaque of atheroma juts into the lumen of the artery. The silky smooth lining of the arteries is mechanically damaged by the pulsatile force of blood as it moves through arteries that are elastic and are constantly moving in pulsation. With every pulse wave, the arterial wall yields and is stretched; over many years some damage must occur. The damage is partially repaired by small blood particles (platelets), which clump together and plug the damaged surface. These platelet plugs form a temporary patch, just like the plug of coagulated blood you see when you nick yourself and a very small clot forms. In the coronary arteries or aorta, small clots are commonly formed on the lining.[4] Presumably these are involved in the repair of injuries to the smooth lining of the arteries. These small blood clots are somehow welded into the lining as hard thickened areas (fibrous plaques). The artery is trying to strengthen its wall in this repair job.

Fibrous tissue is formed from special cells that are produced everywhere in the body when a repair job is needed; for example, a few days after a large cut or surgical wound is stitched, fibrous tissue cells move in to form a bridge, which transforms over the next weeks into a scar. Fibrous tissue therefore forms scars. Some scars are smooth; some are bumpy

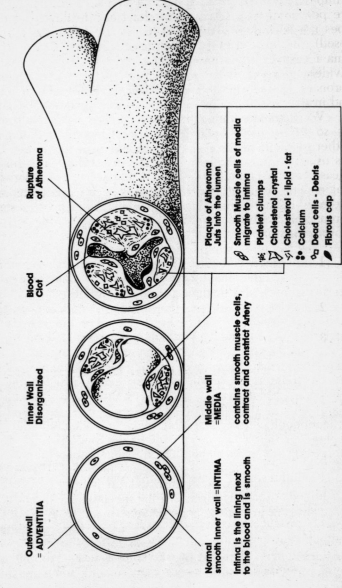

## Figure 1-4.  Atherosclerosis of Artery

Outerwall
= ADVENTITIA

Inner Wall
Disorganized

Blood
Clot

Rupture
of Atheroma

Middle wall
= MEDIA

contains smooth muscle cells,
contract and constrict Artery

Normal
smooth inner wall = INTIMA

Intima is the lining next
to the blood and is smooth

Plaque of Atheroma
Juts into the lumen

Smooth Muscle cells of media
migrate to Intima

Platelet clumps

Cholesterol crystal

Cholesterol - lipid - fat

Calcium

Dead cells - Debris

Fibrous cap

and rough. So are the plaques of atheroma sometimes smooth, bumpy, large, rough, and even ulcerated. These tough scars are perhaps nature's way of patching and healing, but nature does not always win. Because the vessel wall gets hard (sclerosed), the term used for the disease is atherosclerosis. Atheroma is usually most prominent in the abdominal aorta as it divides to form the vessels to the pelvis and lower limbs, in the coronary arteries, in the carotid arteries to the neck and brain, and in the vessels of the lower limbs (Figure 1-5).

When the coronary arteries are involved with atherosclerosis so as to cause symptoms, many doctors use the term "atherosclerotic heart disease" or "ischemic heart disease." Others use the term "coronary heart disease," and since this term is easier for the public to understand, I will use it in this book. Angina and heart attacks are the two main manifestations of coronary heart disease. A heart attack is due to blockage of a coronary artery, and such a blockage is usually due to one or more of the following:

1. A blood clot forms on a plaque of atheroma (Figure 1-4). The plaque may be fissured (ulcerated or ruptured), and this often leads to clotting.

2. A large plaque of atheroma nearly completely blocks the artery.

3. Small blood particles (platelets) may stick to the surface of the plaque in clumps similar to sludge in pipes. The clumped material may dislodge and be wafted downstream by the blood and may block a smaller artery.

4. A coronary artery may go into spasm, especially at the site of a plaque, blocking the vessel for a few minutes or a few hours (coronary artery spasm).

5. An increase in adrenaline can be produced under the influence of stress or other inciting factors and can cause clumping of platelets that may lead to clot formation. Excess adrenaline from any source can also produce electrical disturbances in the heart, especially ventricular fibrillation. In fibrillation the heart muscle stops contracting and quivers; therefore no blood is pumped, i.e., a cardiac arrest.

## Figure 1-5. Heart and Arteries

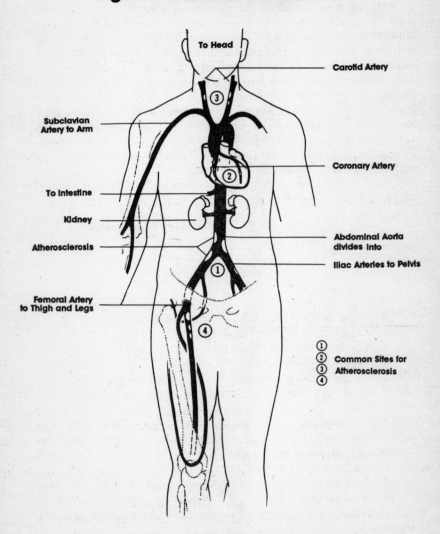

Note that the factors are largely mechanical, influenced by many unknown variables present in the blood during its turbulent flow through the narrowed arteries. Because of the varied nature of the blockage, we cannot speak of complete prevention of heart attacks by any single nondrug treatment or by any single drug. We can try to influence the mechanical factors and hope to reduce their occurrence or recurrence by paying attention to the prevention of blood clotting and by modification of the so-called risk factors. Over the past fifty years, cardiologists and scientists alike have studied atherosclerosis with little emphasis on the clotting of blood—or its prevention. Current books on how to prevent heart attacks dwell mainly on the prevention of atherosclerosis by asking you to modify three major risk factors: cholesterol, hypertension, and smoking. These so-called risk factors only minimally influence the clotting of blood. Thus it is not surprising to this author that the epidemic of deaths from heart attack continues. However, I will deal with identification and management of the conventional risk factors because my views are in keeping with the body of scientific evidence, which has demonstrated that the three factors are important. Then I will discuss blood clots and ventricular fibrillation.

## WHAT ARE RISK FACTORS?

The identification of factors that increase the risk of heart attack has been made possible by various population studies, including the well-known Framingham Study. The statistical correlation has been so consistent as to enable rsearchers to state with confidence that high blood pressure (hypertension), a high blood cholesterol, and cigarette smoking are major risk factors and, if present, increase your probability of having a fatal or nonfatal heart attack or stroke.

The risk factors can be subdivided into three groups. Group I consists of factors over which we have no control. Group II includes four controllable risk factors. Group III includes other important factors.

## GROUP I: UNCONTROLLABLE RISK FACTORS

1. **Heredity.** A strong family history of heart attack especially before age fifty increases the risk.
2. **Age.** Risk increases with age, but death by heart attack is more common in patients less than age fifty; therefore, do your best to get past fifty-two.
3. **Sex.** Everyone recognizes that heart attacks are about ten times more common in men than in women in the thirty to forty-five age group.

## GROUP II: CONTROLLABLE RISK FACTORS

1. Hypertension
2. High blood cholesterol
3. Cigarette smoking
4. Stress

## GROUP III: OTHER FACTORS OF IMPORTANCE

1. Diabetes
2. Sedentary lifestyle, lack of exercise
3. Strenuous unaccustomed exertion
4. Obesity
5. Type A personality

If you are a male over age thirty-five and have one of the four major risk factors—hypertension, high blood cholesterol, cigarette smoking or stress—your chance of having a heart attack doubles. Two risk factors increases your risk to more than three times that of a person with no risk factors. If you have all four, your risk increases to about seven times. However, no one can predict with any degree of certainty who is going to have a heart attack. Some people are just plain lucky. They have the correct genes; "they chose their parents." They disobey all the rules: two eggs and two packets of cigarettes daily from age twenty to seventy-five, never exercise, and lead a stressful life and yet never have a heart attack. People of this type fortunately have blood pressures that are on the low side of normal (100 to 115 systolic). If your blood pressure is low (less than 110/80), and you are average or slightly underweight and your parents both lived to beyond seventy-five, you are on the right side of the track.

# CHAPTER 2

# IS CHOLESTEROL IMPORTANT AGAIN?

The importance of an elevated blood cholesterol in the causation of atherosclerosis and a subsequent heart attack has been a controversial issue for more than forty years. Therefore, advice to patients has often been halfhearted. Until recently we were not able to put the blame firmly on cholesterol and convince our colleagues and patients. We were missing the key piece of scientific evidence—that lowering of elevated blood cholesterol in humans prevents fatal or nonfatal heart attacks.

In 1984, the Lipid Research Clinics Program[5] reported the results of a successful trial that they conducted in the United States over a period of ten years at a cost of $150 million. The trial showed that a reduction in blood cholesterol resulted in a small but significant reduction in fatal and nonfatal heart attacks.

The study was randomized, and scrupulously conducted in many centers in the United States and in two centers in Canada. More than 480,000 men aged thirty-five to fifty-nine were screened to find subjects who had a cholesterol level greater than 265 milligrams per 100 milliliters of blood (mg/dL) but were otherwise healthy and, in particular, had no evidence of heart disease or hypertension. The 3,806 men found suitable for the trial were asked to follow a cholesterol-lowering diet. A random half of the men were given a drug to lower cholesterol (cholestyramine, 24 g daily); the other random half were given an identical-looking but nonmedicinal preparation (placebo). The drug caused an 8 percent lowering of the blood cholesterol.

After follow-up for an average of 7.4 years, there were 187 fatal or nonfatal heart attacks in the controls and 155 in the drug-treated group. Unfortunately, cholestyramine is a powder that is mixed with fruit juice and is unpleasant to taste. Patients do not comply with taking it two or three times daily, and it is not surprising that the reduction in cholesterol was 8 percent rather than an expected 25 percent. Nevertheless, the study shows that lowering of cholesterol by a special drug reduces the occurrence of heart attack. Thus a reduction of blood cholesterol by diet should have a similar good effect.

A diet that will lower blood cholesterol by 10 percent is feasible. This has been well tested and is expected to reduce the incidence of fatal and nonfatal heart attacks. A clinical trial using a low cholesterol diet alone will never be done since it will require vast numbers of patients and medical manpower at a cost of more than $1 billion. Futhermore, it is difficult to prevent the controlled patients from dieting when they recognize that it may be helpful; therefore exact scientific evaluation is impossible.

*What is a normal blood cholesterol, and when does the level produce a risk of coronary heart disease?*

Blood cholesterol is not necessarily high, i.e., greater than 265 milligrams, in those who have heart attacks. In fact, most heart attacks occur in individuals with blood cholesterol around the average 220 to 250 mg/dL. You may understand this by noting that in the Lipid Study described, only 3,806 men with a blood cholesterol greater than 265 mg could be found from a screen of 480,000. The remainder had cholesterol blood levels of less than 265 mg and likely 200 to 250 mg.

Laboratories in North America report a normal cholesterol as being between 150 and 250 mg. But it is now established that individuals with so-called normal cholesterol in the range of 220 to 250 are at increased risk, and heart attacks are common in individuals with such levels. A blood cholesterol of 220 to 250 mg is considered high by world standards and can no longer be considered normal. Most doctors now talk about an optimal level, i.e., a level that can be considered safe. I agree with experts who state that a cholesterol less than 200 mg is optimal, and heart attacks are uncommon in individuals with a cholesterol less than 200 mg.

If we wait to treat patients with a cholesterol level greater than 250 mg with nondrug therapy, we will be excluding more than 80 percent of the population who are at high risk. To reemphasize, most heart attacks in North America occur in subjects with a blood cholesterol between 220 and 260 mg, that is, in a range often unnoticed by your doctor. If your cholesterol is less than 190 mg, you obviously deal with cholesterol by your own natural process. You are among the fortunate, and no dietary modification is necessary.

Studies that support the cholesterol hypothesis include the following:

1. In Norway, a five-year study of more than 1,000 men aged forty to forty-nine showed a reduced incidence of coronary heart disease in those whose blood cholesterol was lowered.[6]

2. The Seven Countries Study included more than 12,000 men from Finland, Greece, Italy, Netherlands, Japan, the United States, and Yugoslavia.[7] The Finns had the highest intake of saturated fat, the highest blood cholesterol levels (greater than 280 mg), and the highest number of fatal and nonfatal heart attacks, about 900 per 100,000. The Japanese with an average blood cholesterol of 140 mg had the lowest heart attack death rate of 102 per 100,000. The United States with an average of 220 mg/dL had a heart attack death rate of 670 per 100,000. The death rate was also low in Greece and Italy. Japanese who immigrate to the United States and are accustomed to an American diet have an incidence of coronary heart disease ten times that of their countrymen in Japan.

3. The Framingham Study has contributed good evidence to support the view that a high blood cholesterol greatly increases the risk of developing coronary heart disease.[8]

4. People who have a rare inherited defect that prevents the body from getting rid of cholesterol may have blood cholesterol levels as high as 1,000 mg from early childhood. These individuals may have heart attacks in their teens or before age thirty. These patients develop cholesterol-containing lumps and bumps especially on the knees, elbows, and tendons of the wrists

and the Achilles' tendon. Fortunately the condition is very rare.

5.  Rabbits fed a high-cholesterol diet develop severe atherosclerosis of the aorta and coronary arteries; similar lesions can be produced in monkeys and swine. The atheromatous lesions partially regress with reduction of the blood cholesterol in animals.

6.  A recent Heart, Lung and Blood Institute Study showed that a reduction in blood cholesterol by the drug cholestyramine tends to prevent enlargement of atherosclerotic plaques in man.[9]

In order to understand the changes that may be required in your diet, you must understand the following terms: cholesterol, lipoproteins, low-density lipoprotein (LDL) cholesterol, high-density lipoprotein (HDL) cholesterol, triglycerides, saturated fats, unsaturated fats, and polyunsaturated fats.

## CHOLESTEROL

Some of the cholesterol in the blood is derived from the food you eat, but the major part, greater than 70 percent, is manufactured in the liver, mainly from saturated fats. Thus, if we had no cholesterol in the diet, the liver would manufacture more cholesterol to compensate. Cholesterol is an essential part of the fatty sheath that insulates nerves, the outer membrane of cells, and a component of chemicals that include steroids (cortisone) and sex hormones such as androgens and estrogens. Some excess cholesterol is excreted in the bile.

Cholesterol is present only in foods of animal origin, in particular, eggs, milk, butter, cheese, and meats, and a very high concentration is present in gland meats, such as liver, brain, kidney, heart, and sweetbread. Plant-based foods such as vegetables, fruits, grains, and beans contain no cholesterol.

Cholesterol is a fat (lipid) that is insoluble in water and does not get into the solution of the blood. Cholesterol absorbed by the intestine or released from the liver into the blood stream does not circulate freely in solution, but is attached to a protein carrier, forming a molecule called a lipoprotein. Imagine cholesterol being transported in its own boxcar called a low-density lipoprotein; therefore, the term "low-density lipoprotein (LDL) cholesterol."

There are several lipoproteins that vary in size and density; the smaller the size, the higher the density. There is also a high-density lipoprotein (HDL) cholesterol. When your doctor states that your cholesterol is 250 mg, he or she is giving you the total amount of cholesterol in the blood, which includes, for example, about 200 mg of LDL cholesterol and about 50 mg of HDL cholesterol. The total figure is not broken down unless specifically requested by the doctor.

## Low-Density Lipoprotein ("Bad") Cholesterol

The LDL is small and dense and contains most of the cholesterol that is transported to cells. The higher the level of LDL cholesterol in the blood, the greater the risk of coronary heart disease; thus, the term "bad" cholesterol. About 75 percent of the blood cholesterol is carried as LDL cholesterol.

## High-Density Lipoprotein ("Good") Cholesterol

Recently much interest has been focused on high-density lipoprotein cholesterol, so called because it is very small in size and very high in density. It carries the cholesterol away from body cells such as the lining of arteries, thereby helping to keep the artery wall clean; thus the term "good" cholesterol. About 25 percent of the blood cholesterol is carried as HDL cholesterol. People with high levels of HDL cholesterol, greater than 60 mg, appear to live longer and have less coronary heart disease. People with levels less than 30 mg have an increased risk of coronary heart disease. However, do not be alarmed if your HDL is less than 30 mg. These findings need to be substantiated by further scientific studies. It is not clear why some people should have high and others very low values.

Females and males prior to puberty have the same cholesterol levels. Boys, however, at puberty have about a 20 percent drop in HDL and a rise in LDL cholesterol. The decrease in HDL cholesterol may be due to an increase in androgens. In men the HDL level stays fairly constant up to age fifty then starts to rise steeply between fifty to sixty-five. It is possible that this rise might be due to a decrease of androgens, which occurs during the male climacteric period, whereas in women there is a gradual rise in HDL cholesterol from age twenty-five onwards. Women are believed to be protected to postmenopause by this increase in HDL and by their hormonal status. Why women are protected from coronary heart disease until the menopause and yet not protected from strokes is not easily explained, especially if atherosclerosis is the basis of both diseases.

We will now look at the relationship between HDL cholesterol and population groups, foods, alcohol, exercise, and drugs.

1.  Population groups. The Japanese, Eskimo men, and the black population in England, Jamaica, South Africa, and the United States appear to have higher HDL cholesterol levels than whites.[10] The exact reason for this finding is unknown; it may be due to a combination of genetic or environmental factors and diet.

2.  Foods. A low-saturated fat, low-cholesterol diet modified to be acceptable to patients does not cause a change in HDL cholesterol levels. However, a very low-saturated fat diet causes a reduction in HDL cholesterol. A high-carbohydrate diet produces a mild fall in HDL cholesterol.[10] A vegetarian diet may cause a slight decrease in HDL and this may be due to an increased carbohydrate intake. Obesity is associated with a low-HDL level and patients with very high triglyceride levels often have low HDL levels.

3.  Exercise. Daily strenuous exercise such as long-distance running can increase HDL levels by 5 to 10 percent. It is unfortunate that moderate exercise five times weekly to produce the training effect (cardiovascular fitness) does not significantly increase HDL levels.[10] No one has documented that a rise in HDL cholesterol from 40 to 45 to 48 mg reduces cardiovascular risk. There

appears to be a clear difference between 30 and 60 mg with regards to risk. Therefore, I do not advise you to take up long-distance running to elevate your levels by 5 to 10 percent. Jogging one to three miles daily or every other day will produce the training effect but appears to have little or an inconsistent effect on HDL levels.

4.   Drugs. There are a few drugs that alter HDL levels slightly; however, they are considered only experimental at this stage. The pharmaceutical companies are certainly busy in this area trying to develop such compounds, but they will require several years of testing, especially with regards to safety.

A reasonable indication of the risk of coronary heart disease can be deduced from the amount of HDL cholesterol relative to the total cholesterol. For example, if your total cholesterol is 240 mg and HDL cholesterol 60 mg, the percent of HDL cholesterol will be $60 \div 240 \times 100 = 25$ percent. This puts you into the below-average coronary heart disease risk (i.e., good risk). The risk categories are as follows:

| CORONARY HEART DISEASE RISK | PERCENT HDL CHOLESTEROL |
|---|---|
| Lowest risk group | Greater than 28 |
| Below average | 22–28 |
| Average | 15–22 |
| High | 7–15 |
| Highest | Less than 7 |

## Very Low-Density Lipoprotein (VLDL)

The VLDL is very large and low in density. VLDL transports triglycerides, which are used mainly as a fuel; for example, in exercising muscle. The evidence linking elevated blood triglyceride levels with coronary heart disease is very weak and unclear. Thus, an elevated blood triglyceride level alone is not of importance.

## Genetic Defect and Cholesterol

In very rare cases, marked elevation of cholesterol (600 to 1200 mg) is caused by a genetic defect. A receptor on the surface of cells (LDL receptors) removes LDL cholesterol from the blood. These receptors are genetically deficient in approximately 1 in 1,000 Americans and cause a marked increase in blood cholesterol. Deposits of cholesterol (xanthomas) occur as creamy yellow streaks under the eyelids, or on the Achilles' tendon, the back of the hands and over bony prominences such as the knees and elbows. These people may have coronary heart disease in childhood or early adult life, but fortunately, the condition is very rare. Racial differences may determine the number of LDL receptors, and thus the ability to remove LDL cholesterol gradually from the blood stream is affected. About 20 percent of the population have all the luck. They can eat a high-cholesterol, saturated fat diet and violate all rules and yet never get significant coronary heart disease and live beyond seventy-five.

## Blood Tests

The blood cholesterol measurement gives the total blood cholesterol, i.e., LDL cholesterol plus HDL cholesterol. The food you eat does not have an immediate effect on your blood cholesterol and HDL cholesterol measurements so fasting is not necessary for their determination. Triglyceride is not an independent risk factor and therefore widespread screening for elevated triglyceride is not warranted. It is also an expensive investigation. If your doctor thinks that triglyceride determination is necessary, you must fast for fourteen hours before the blood is taken. Blood tests for glucose, diabetic check, or triglycerides are the only tests for which it is necessary to fast for twelve to fourteen hours before the test. Determination of LDL cholesterol is not done routinely, because it is a difficult, time-consuming, and expensive technique. It is easier for a doctor to relate the risk of coronary heart disease with total blood cholesterol, since the statistics have been available for the past thirty years.

## SATURATED AND UNSATURATED FATS

All animal fat is saturated and solid at normal room temperatures. The degree of hydrogenation of a fat determines how solid and saturated it is. Saturated fats are broken down in the body and increase the blood cholesterol. Therefore the most effective dietary method of lowering blood cholesterol is to reduce intake of saturated fats. Vegetable fats are unsaturated and almost all are liquid at room temperatures. There are three vegetable oils that you must avoid: coconut oil, palm oil, and peanut oil. Coconut oil contains a high amount of saturated fat and is commonly used for cooking in several countries. It is also used in North America in nondairy cream substitutes, for example, coffee cream. Therefore, beware of coffee cream substitutes. Palm oil contains significant amounts of saturated fat, and peanut oil, though mainly unsaturated, has certain fatty acids that produce plaques of atheroma in animals. The only vegetable that contains a little saturated fat is the avocado; therefore, low-cholesterol, low-fat diets, often recommend that you avoid avocados. However, you will note from Table 2-1 that although a large avocado contains a significant amount of fat, only a little of it is saturated, and no cholesterol is present. Therefore, one avocado used twice weekly is an excellent food, especially if a high potassium intake is required.

## TABLE 2-1 SATURATED FAT, POLYUNSATURATED AND CHOLESTEROL CONTENT OF FOODS

| * ITEM | CHOLES-TEROL | TOTAL FAT | SATURATED FAT | NOT RECOM-MENDED | ** RECOM-MENDED | USE SPARINGLY |
|---|---|---|---|---|---|---|
| | mg | g | g | | | |
| **MEATS** | | | | | | |
| beef liver | 395 | 10 | 3 | X | | |
| kidney | 725 | 11 | 4 | X | | |
| sweetbread | 420 | 21 | - | X | | |
| lean beef | 82 | 5 | 2 | | ** | |
| roast beef | | | | | | |
| eg. rib | 85 | 33 | 14 | X | | ¢ |
| rump | 85 | 21 | 9 | X | | |
| stewing | 82 | 27 | 11 | X | | ¢ |
| " lean | 82 | 9 | 4 | | ** | |
| ground | 85 | 18 | 8 | X | | ¢ |
| steak | | | | | | |
| sirloin | 85 | 25 | 10 | X | | ¢ |
| " lean | 85 | 5 | 2 | | ** | |
| veal | 90 | 12 | 5 | | ** | |
| lamb, lean | 90 | 7 | 4 | | | ¢ |
| chop & fat | 110 | 33 | 18 | X | | |
| ham | | | | | | |
| fat roasted | 80 | 28 | 7 | X | | |
| boiled | | | | | | |
| sliced | 80 | 18 | 5 | | | ¢ |
| pork chop | 80 | 30 | 12 | X | | |
| chicken | | | | | | |
| breast & | | | | | | |
| skin | 72 | 6 | 1 | | ** | |
| drumstick | | | | | | |
| fried | 80 | 9 | 2 | | ** | |
| turkey | 80 | 5 | 2 | | ** | |
| | | | | | | |
| **FISH** | | | | | | |
| sole | 45 | 1 | trace | | ** | |
| trout | 50 | 13 | 3 | | ** | |
| tuna | 60 | 7 | 2 | | ** | |
| salmon | | | | | | |
| fresh | 42 | 7 | 1 | | ** | |
| canned | 32 | 11 | 2 | | ** | |
| mackerel | 85 | 10 | 2 | | ** | |

* Quantity is 3 oz, 90 g unless specified, 15 ml = one tablespoon.
** Foods recommended contain less than 5 g saturated fat per 3 oz.

## TABLE 2-1 SATURATED FAT, POLYUNSATURATED AND CHOLESTEROL CONTENT OF FOODS

| *<br>ITEM | CHOLES-<br>TEROL | TOTAL<br>FAT | SATURATED<br>FAT | NOT<br>RECOM-<br>MENDED | **<br>RECOM-<br>MENDED | USE<br>SPARINGLY |
|---|---|---|---|---|---|---|
| | mg | g | g | | | |
| halibut | 54 | 6 | trace | | ** | |
| crabmeat | 91 | 1 | trace | | | ¢ |
| shrimps | 130 | 1 | trace | | | ¢ |
| lobster | 80 | 1 | trace | | | ¢ |
| 450 g | | | | | | |
| 30 ml butter | 460 | 25 | 16 | X | | |
| egg 50 g | 275 | 6 | 2 | | | ¢ |
| substitute | 0 | 0 | 0 | | ** | |
| buttermilk† | 10 | 2 | 1 | | | |
| yogurt† | | | | | | |
| (250 ml) | 16 | 3 | 2 | | ** | |

## TABLE 2-1 SATURATED FAT, POLYUNSATURATED AND CHOLESTEROL CONTENT OF FOODS

| *<br>ITEM | CHOLES-<br>TEROL | TOTAL<br>FAT | SATURATED<br>FAT | POLY-<br>UNSAT-<br>URATED | NOT<br>RECOM. | **<br>RECOM. | USE<br>SPAR-<br>INGLY |
|---|---|---|---|---|---|---|---|
| | mg | g | g | | | | |
| whole milk | | | | | | | |
| 250 ml | 35 | 9 | 5 | | | | ¢ |
| 2% | 20 | 5 | 3 | | | ** | |
| skim milk | trace | trace | trace | | | ** | |
| avocados | | | | | | | |
| ⅓ of | 0 | 11 | 2 | | | ** | |
| California | | | | | | | |
| ⅓ Florida | 0 | 6.5 | 1 | | | ** | |

* Quantity is 3 oz, 90 g unless specified, 15 ml = one tablespoonful.
** Foods Recommended contain less than 5 g saturated fat per 3 oz
† Low-fat milk, 2%.

## TABLE 2-1 SATURATED FAT, POLYUNSATURATED AND CHOLESTEROL CONTENT OF FOODS CONTINUED

| * ITEM | CHOLES-TEROL | TOTAL FAT | SATURATED FAT | POLY-UNSAT-URATED | NOT RECOM. | ** RECOM. | USE SPAR-INGLY |
|---|---|---|---|---|---|---|---|
| | mg | g | g | | | | |
| ice cream | | | | | | | |
| vanilla reg. 125 ml | 32 | 8 | 5 | | | | ¢ |
| rich 125 ml | 46 | 12 | 8 | | X | | |
| butter*** | 30 | 11 | 7 | trace | | | ¢ |
| lard*** | 12 | 13 | 5 | 1 | X | | |
| OILS*** | | | | | | | |
| corn oil | 0 | 14 | 1 | 7 | | **- | |
| rapeseed | 0 | 14 | 1 | 3 | | | ¢ |
| safflower | 0 | 13 | 1 | 10 | | ** | |
| sunflower | 0 | 14 | 1 | 9 | | ** | |
| soyabean | 0 | 14 | 2 | 7 | | ** | |
| coconut | 0 | 14 | 12 | .2 | X | | |
| palm | 0 | 7 | | .2 | X | | |
| olive | 0 | 14 | 2 | 1 | | | ¢ |
| peanut | | 14 | 2 | 4 | X | | |
| cheese 1 oz | | | | | | | |
| brick | 27 | 8 | 6 | trace | | | ¢ |
| blue | 24 | | | " | | ¢ | |
| cheddar | 30 | 10 | 6 | " | | | ¢ |
| cottage† | 2 | .6 | .5 | " | | ** | |
| skim milk | | | | | | | |
| processed 1 oz 30 g | 0 | trace | trace | trace | | ** | |
| almonds | 0 | 16 | 1 | 3 | | ** | |
| brazil nuts | 0 | 22 | 5 | 8 | X | | |
| cashews | 0 | 13 | 3 | 2 | X | | |
| coconut | 0 | 13 | 11 | trace | X | | |
| peanuts | 0 | 17 | 3 | 4 | X | | |
| peanut butter*** | 0 | 7.5 | 1.5 | 2 | X | | |
| pecans | 0 | 21 | 2 | 5 | | | ¢ |
| walnuts | 0 | 19 | 2 | 11 | | ** | |

* Quantity is 3 oz, 90 g unless specified, 15 ml = one tablespoonful.
** Foods Recommended contain less than 5 g saturated fat per 3 oz
† Low-fat milk, 2%.

## OTHER FOODS

Several foods, especially various fatty acids, show great promise in certain population groups in causing a reduction in cholesterol, blood-clotting factors, and atherosclerosis. These foods include:

1.  Fish oils containing omega-3 fatty acids, especially eicosapentaenoic acid.[11] This acid, present in the diet of Eskimos and fish-eating Japanese, prevents clumping of platelets and has favorable effects on the blood-clotting system.[12][13]
2.  Onions and garlic. Sixty milligrams of fried or boiled onions have been shown to normalize the increase in blood cholesterol and clotting properties of the blood induced by a fatty meal.[14] Garlic appears to have a similar favorable effect. Other plant materials are being investigated.
3.  Soybean-derived products, which prevent the development of atheroma and cause a decrease in the size of plaques in experimental animals.

It is important to note that many recipes developed for weight reduction diets tend to cut out carbohydrate foods in order to decrease weight and may even introduce foods that increase blood clotting and cholesterol. Therefore, be careful in choosing "popular" weight reduction diets. I advise you to consult Table 2-1 and the instructions given under "Sensible Heart Diet."

## DIETS

Diets to reduce atherosclerosis or heart attacks must be individualized since each family has different eating habits. I emphasize that special recipes and diet sheets may be misleading, and difficult to follow for a lifetime. Therefore, I do not recommend recipes or diet sheets in this book. Any person requiring a diet may consult Table 2-1, or similar information.

It is recommended that you use foods that contain a low amount of saturated fat and cholesterol, and make an effort to increase the intake of polyunsaturated fat and foods that have a favorable effect on blood clotting. Reduction in the intake of cholesterol alone is not sufficient since saturated fat is converted into cholesterol in the body. Therefore, you must reduce your saturated fat intake. The recommendation made by the American Heart Association and Senate Committee in 1978 and followed by many Americans is as follows:

> Total fat intake should be reduced from the average 40 percent of calories to 30 percent. Polyunsaturated fat should provide up to 10 percent of calories and the polyunsaturated fat to saturated fat (P/S) ratio should be about 1. Carbohydrate intake to be increased from an average of about 45 percent to 55 percent to maintain average body weight, and protein to remain about 12 to 14 percent. It is believed that this reduction in dietary fat intake as well as the cessation of smoking by many Americans has provided a significant decline in the incidence of coronary heart disease mortality.

However, the United Kingdom has not shared in the slight decline in mortality that has been experienced in Australia, Belgium, Canada, Finland, Norway, and the United States. Scotland has moved up in the world league table of coronary deaths to second for men and first for women, and Northern Ireland has moved to third for men and second for women.[15] In the United Kingdom, fat intake has remained the same for the past thirty years at about 40 percent of food energy, and even increased between 1974 to 1982 to 41 percent of food energy. Consequently in mid-1984, the Department of Health and Social Security made the following recommendations to physicians and the general public in the United Kingdom: Reduce the total fat intake to 35 percent of food energy, with saturated fats 11%. Increase the P/S ratio from the present 0.27 to about 0.45. The intake of polyunsaturated acids presently at 5 percent of food energy should reach 7 percent, which is less than the American and World Health Organization's suggestion of 10 percent. The U.K. panel claims that the effects on the population of a P/S ratio of 1.0 and beyond are unknown.[15] However, individuals who are considered to have a high risk of developing coronary heart disease are advised to cut fats to 30 percent of food energy with saturated fats contributing no more than 10 percent, i.e., identical to the recommendation in the United States. Thus, there is consensus on both sides of the Atlantic.

## SENSIBLE HEART DIET

Consult Table 2-1 and follow the advice given in A, B, and C below. This will fulfill the recommendation of fat intake to be 30 percent of food energy. You will receive enough polyunsaturated fat and protein without having to do complicated calculations. The American Heart Association Prudent Diet gives similar recommendations.[16]

These recommendations do not strictly apply if your blood cholesterol is less than 200 mg/dL since you obviously deal with cholesterol by your own natural process. Foods with a high salt (sodium) content should be avoided or used sparingly. See Table 2-2 "List of Foods with Comparative Sodium Content."

**A.**  Do Not Use the Following Foods:
1. Organ meats such as liver, kidney, sweetbreads, heart, or brain.
2. Meat fat, heavily marbled steaks, mutton, salt pork, or duck.
3. Whole milk or whole milk products, cream, lard, and nonvegetable margarine.
4. Coconut oil or products containing coconut oil such as nondairy coffee cream substitutes, palm oil, and peanut oil or peanut butter.

**B.**  Use the Following Foods Sparingly and in Small Amounts:
1. Roast beef, luncheon meats, bacon, sausages, hamburger, and spare ribs.
2. Butter, egg yolk, cheese made from whole milk or cream, pies, chocolate pudding, whole milk pudding, and ice cream.

3. Lobster, which has a high cholesterol content and is often served with abundant butter; therefore use sparingly.
4. Peanuts, cashew, and brazil nuts.

C.   Use the Following Recommended Foods Often:
1. All vegetables, including lentils and split peas, which are rich in protein and fiber; fruits including avocado despite its very small saturated fat content. However, do not "overindulge" in vegetables containing a high content of Vitamin K such as broccoli, alfalfa, turnip greens, squash, and lettuce, because an increase in Vitamin K intake may increase clot formation.
2. Fish of all types even when described as fatty fish contains little saturated fat but has an abundance of special polyunsaturated fat that protects the arteries. Shrimps are not as bad as claimed, provided they are not fried in a batter and only used occasionally. Remember, any food fried in batter increases the saturated fat content.
3. Poultry, chicken breast, or turkey, which, when cooked with the skin taken off, contains very little saturated fat or cholesterol. You must cut fat from meat including chicken before cooking.
4. Lean beef or veal.
5. Fat and oils. Polyunsaturated vegetable oils such as safflower oil, sunflower seed oil, corn oil, soybean oil, sesame seed, and cotton seed oil should be used for cooking, and polyunsaturated margarine to be used as much as possible in place of butter. It is advisable to use butter sparingly when eating outside your home and to use a polyunsaturated margarine at home.
6. Carbohydrates (sugars and starchy foods) such as bread or other flour products, potato, and rice to maintain normal body weight.
7. Onions and garlic. Use garlic powder, not garlic salt, which has a high sodium content (see Table 2-2).
8. Almonds and walnuts, which are high in polyunsaturated fat content and are thus recommended.

You need a low–saturated fat, low-cholesterol diet; therefore, choose foods known to have low saturated fat and moderate to low cholesterol content. In this respect, the foods listed in Table 2-1 are recommended if a three-ounce portion contains less than five grams of saturated fat. The cholesterol content of most meats and poultry is similar and not excessive; therefore, no recommendations are based on the cholesterol content of these foods except for glandular meats, which are very high in cholesterol content and must be avoided (see Table 2-1). Despite their high cholesterol content, eggs are an excellent and readily available source of nutrients. One egg can be used two or three times weekly, and at other times, an egg substitute can be used.

## DRUGS TO REDUCE BLOOD CHOLESTEROL

Drugs are rarely used because they reduce cholesterol only 8 to 20 percent. In addition, some are unpleasant to taste and others have serious side effects. Fortunately there are a few promising new drugs, and manufacturers are screening several compounds.

In patients under age sixty, if the blood cholesterol remains greater than 260 mg/dL (6.72 millimoles per litre) mmoL/L, despite a twelve-month trial of adequate diet, drugs may be utilized. Drug treatment in patients over sixty is of no value. The decision to treat with drugs will depend on your doctor's evaluation of:

1. The importance of the 1984 results of the Lipid Research Clinics Study, in which the drug cholestyramine used in healthy individuals with a cholesterol greater than 260 mg caused a reduction in coronary heart disease events, i.e., fatal and nonfatal heart attacks.[5]
2. Your other risk factors: presence of hypertension, smoking, and a family history of heart attacks before age fifty.

## TABLE 2-2 LIST OF FOODS WITH COMPARATIVE SODIUM (Na) CONTENT

| FOOD | PORTION | MG SODIUM |
|---|---|---|
| Bouillon | 1 cube | 900 |
| Bacon back | 1 slice | 500 |
| Bacon side (fried crisp) | 1 slice | 75 |
| Beef (lean, cooked) | 3 oz (90 g) | 60 |
| Garlic salt | 1 teaspoon (15 ml) | 2000 |
| Garlic powder | 1 teaspoon | 2 |
| Ham cured | 3 oz (90 g) | 1000 |
| Ham fresh cooked | 3 oz | 100 |
| Ketchup | 1 tablespoon | 150 |
| Milk pudding instant whole | 1 cup (250 ml) | 1000 |
| Meat tenderized regular | 1 teaspoon | 2000 |
| Meat tenderized low Na | 1 teaspoon | 2 |
| Olive green | 1 | 100 |
| Pickle dill | Large (10 × 4½ cm) | 1900 |
| Peanuts dry roasted | 1 cup | 1000 |
| Peanuts dry roasted (unsalted) | 1 cup | 10 |
| Wieners | 1 (50 g) | 500 |

### CANNED FOODS

| | | |
|---|---|---|
| Carrots | 4 oz | 400 |
| (Carrots raw) | | 40 |
| Corn whole kernel | 1 cup | 400 |
| (Corn frozen) | 1 cup | 10 |
| Corn beef cooked | 4 oz | 1000 |
| Crab | 3 oz | 900 |
| Peas cooked green | 1 cup | 5 |
| Shrimp | 3 oz | 2000 |
| Salmon salt added | 3 oz | 500 |
| Salmon no salt added | 3 oz | 50 |
| Soups (majority) | 1 cup (250 ml) | 1000 |
| Sauerkraut | 1 cup (250 ml) | 1800 |

### SALAD DRESSING

| | | |
|---|---|---|
| Blue cheese | 15 ml | 160 |
| French regular | 15 ml | 200 |
| Italian | 15 ml | 110 |
| Oil and Vinegar | 15 ml | 1 |
| Thousand Island | 15 ml | 90 |

### FAST FOOD

| | | |
|---|---|---|
| Chopped steak | one portion | 1000 |
| Fried chicken | 3 piece dinner | 2000 |
| Fish & chips | one portion | 1000 |
| Hamburger | double | 1000 |
| Roast beef sandwich | one | 1000 |
| Pizza | one medium | 1000 |

## Cholestyramine

Supplied: Powder in packets or in cans with a scoop.

Dosage: 12 to 24 grams (g) daily in liquid a half hour before to a half hour after meals. Start with 4 g (one scoop) twice daily for one week, then 4 g three times daily for one month and if necessary thereafter increase to 8 g three times daily.

Cholestyramine and colestipol are not absorbed from the gut and act by binding bile salts in the intestine. This action causes the liver to increase the conversion of cholesterol to bile acids, which are excreted in the bile.

Side effects include constipation, nausea, bloating, gas, abdominal cramps, and unpleasant taste. High doses taken for several years can cause poor absorption of certain vitamins. The drugs may interfere with the absorption of digoxin and blood thinners (anticoagulants). Your doctor will decide when to use this potentially useful drug. Usually the patient is under age fifty-five and the blood cholesterol is greater than 260 mg despite a six-month trial of diet.

## Colestipol

Supplied: Powder.

Dosage: 12 to 30 g daily in liquid taken a half hour before to a half hour after meals.

Colestipol is a resin similar to cholestyramine with similar side effects but better patient acceptance.

## Clofibrate

Supplied: Capsules: 0.5 g, 1 g.

Dosage: 0.5 to 1 g twice daily after meals.

The drug can lower triglycerides 10 to 30 percent and cholesterol by 5 to 10 percent; however, the Coronary Drug Project[17] and other studies indicate increased mortality related to the use of the drug. The main indication for the drug is a very rare condition, type III hyperlipoproteinemia, in which the cholesterol is greater than 400 mg and triglycerides greater than 1,000 mg. Fortunately a new drug, gemfibrozil, is of value for this condition. Side effects of clofibrate include nausea, diarrhea, muscle pains, and impotence. Do not use the drug if you have kidney, liver, or gallbladder disease (gallstones).

## D-Thyroxine

D-Thyroxine is not recommended because of several side effects. An increased mortality has been attributed to the drug.[18] A worsening of angina, heart failure, and hypertension do occur.

## Gemfibrozil

Supplied: Capsules: 300 mg (store below 86°F, 30°C).
Dosage: 300 mg taken about a half hour before the morning and the evening meal for one to two weeks, then 600 mg twice daily.
Gemfibrozil is an effective lipid-lowering drug that has a low incidence of adverse effects. The drug is being tested in the five-year Helsinki Heart Study, and results should be available in the late 1980s. It causes a 5 to 10 percent reduction in serum cholesterol, 30 to 40 percent reduction in triglycerides, and a significant increase in HDL ("good") cholesterol, which is very likely to be of value in decreasing risk of coronary heart disease. The drug also appears to have a mild effect in reducing blood clotting without causing bleeding. Side effects are less common than with other drugs listed, and include stomach pain and bloating in less than 5 percent of patients.

## Nicotinic Acid

This drug is not often used because of prominent side effects, which include flushing, itching, nausea, abdominal pain, diarrhea, jaundice, gout, palpitations, and increased blood sugar in diabetics. The drug should not be used if you have a low blood pressure or a heart attack, heart failure, liver disease, stomach ulcer, or diabetes. I do not recommend this drug because of the side effects.

## Probucol

Supplied: Tablets: 250 mg.
Dosage: 500 mg twice daily, with the morning and the evening meal.

Probucol interferes with cholesterol synthesis in the liver and increases excretion of bile acids. The drug is limited by its side effects, which include nausea, flatulence, abdominal pain, diarrhea, palpitations, impotence, and fetid perspiration. The drug unfortunately lowers HDL ("good") cholesterol.

## CONCLUSION

If you are age twenty to sixty, it is advisable to know your total blood cholesterol and HDL ("good") cholesterol. If the values are optimal at age twenty-five, there is no rush to repeat testing until age thirty, then once every one or two years. To do otherwise will strain the finances of people and the state for very little return.

The answer to the question "Is cholesterol important again?" is yes. The evidence is clear. If you can decrease your blood cholesterol to less than 200 mg (5.16 mmol), you can substantially decrease risk of having a heart attack. Patients with a blood cholesterol greater than 280 mg are usually motivated to do something. However, the majority of the North American population age thirty to sixty have a cholesterol in the borderline range of 220 to 250 mg, and in this group the majority of heart attacks occur. They have, therefore, a cholesterol level that is accepted as normal by their doctor, but is clearly abnormal because it causes a high risk of coronary heart disease. I am in agreement with the experts who are concerned with this large population group, and strongly advise you to lower your so-called "normal cholesterol," which is actually undesirably high.

I have given you information so that you can arrange your own Sensible Heart Diet, and I have listed special foods that may prevent blood clots.

# CHAPTER 3

# HIGH BLOOD PRESSURE (HYPERTENSION), A PREVENTABLE RISK FACTOR

High blood pressure (hypertension) is the most preventable risk factor. It is extremely difficult to get the population at risk to discontinue smoking and to reduce consumption of saturated fats and cholesterol. Hypertension, however, can be detected and does respond to nondrug treatment, and where this fails, safe and effective drugs are now available.

Hypertension usually causes no symptoms, but leads to stroke, heart attack, heart failure, kidney damage, and rarely, rupture of an aneurysm. The morbidity and death toll related to this largely asymptomatic disease is colossal and the term "silent killer" is probably appropriate. But this is one time that you can help to prevent the disaster. From age twenty to thirty have your blood pressure checked once yearly, thereafter at least twice yearly.

Hypertension is an important cause of atherosclerosis, and the evidence is solid and not controversial. I will give the following example to illustrate the connection between high blood pressure and atherosclerosis. Atherosclerosis (hardening of the arteries) is never seen in the lung (pulmonary) circulation, except when there is pulmonary hypertension. Large plaques may then develop in the pulmonary arteries that take blood from the right ventricle to the lungs (Figure 1-2). The pulmonary circulation is a low-pressure system in that the pressure in the pulmonary artery is normally about 20 mm systolic and 10 mm diastolic, while the blood pressure in the aorta and its arterial branches (systemic circulation) is normally 100 to 140 mm systolic and 60 to 90 mm diastolic. In individuals with systemic hypertension, the blood pressure in the aorta and branches is commonly 160 to 220 systolic and 95 to 115 mm diastolic, yet the pressure in the pulmonary arteries remains normal and atherosclerosis is never seen. However, if severe pulmonary hypertension develops—for example, a change from 20 mm to 130 mm systolic, and diastolic changes from 10 to 80 mm—plaques of atheroma are then found in the pulmonary artery.

Hypertension therefore causes atherosclerosis. In addition, the walls of the arteries become generally thickened to withstand the increased blood pressure. This leads to further constriction of blood vessels, thereby causing an additional increase in blood pressure.

It is well established that hypertension increases the risk of heart attacks. The risk is considerably increased if there is concomitant high blood cholesterol and/or cigarette smoking. Hypertension causes mechanical damage to the lining of the artery, and cholesterol is drawn into the injured tissues.

While it is difficult to prove that discontinuing smoking and changing the diet reduce cardiovascular risk, there is conclusive scientific evidence that control of hypertension markedly lowers the incidence of stroke, heart failure, and kidney damage, and it is believed to decrease the incidence of fatal and nonfatal heart attacks. Hypertension accelerates atherosclerosis; blockage or rupture of an artery occurs from ten to twenty years earlier than in individuals with normal blood pressures.

The way to measure blood pressure along with nondrug and drug treatment of hypertension are discussed in Chapter 13.

# CHAPTER 4

---

# SMOKING

The latest U.S. Surgeon General's report on smoking and health indicates that, if cigarette smoking were eliminated, about a quarter million lives now lost because of coronary heart disease could be saved yearly in the United States. Each year, lung cancer causes about 80,000 deaths. Smoking causes most cases of lung cancer, which is becoming the leading cause of death from cancer in women.

Nonsmoking men age forty-five to fifty-five are ten times less likely to have a fatal or nonfatal heart attack than heavy smokers. Importantly, the Multiple Risk Factor Intervention Trial showed that men at high risk who stopped smoking had a significant reduction in their mortality.[21]

If you go to the horse races and can pick winners and can follow statistical relationships, you will certainly put your money on cigarette smoking as a major culprit in the causation of fatal and nonfatal heart attacks.

The detrimental effects of cigarette smoking were widely advertised in the mid-1960s, and since then more than 20 million Americans have stopped smoking. However, smoking has increased in teenagers and women, resulting in little change in the overall number of smokers, which remains at about 50 million Americans. Heart attacks are rare in women age thirty-five to forty-five, but in women of this age who use oral contraceptives and smoke, the heart attack rate is definitely increased.

Low-nicotine, low-tar brands or filter cigarettes do not decrease the risk of coronary heart disease,[19] although the risk of lung cancer may be decreased. Filter cigarettes deliver more carbon monoxide and cause a higher incidence of coronary heart disease than do plain cigarettes.[20]

If you cannot quit but can change to a pipe, this will certainly decrease the risk, since studies have shown that pipe and cigar smokers have only a slight increase in cardiac death.[22] However, you must not smoke Cheroot, since a higher risk of heart attacks was found to occur in Danish Cheroot smokers than in cigarette smokers.

## EFFECTS ON COMPONENTS OF CIGARETTE SMOKE

Tobacco smoke contains more than 4,000 components. Some of these are nicotine, carbon monoxide, ammonia, benzene, nitrobenzene, phenol, 2,4 dimethylphenol, acetaldehyde, hydrogen cyanide, toluene, and O-cresol. Most studies have been done on nicotine and various gases, in particular, carbon monoxide (CO). Although the effects of the many constituents of smoke are not understood, the effects of nicotine and CO are well documented.

### Nicotine

Nicotine stimulates the adrenal glands to put out excessive adrenaline and noradrenaline.[23] The higher the nicotine concentration inhaled, the greater the outpouring of adrenaline. If someone puts a gun to your head, you need all the adrenaline and noradrenaline that your adrenals and nerves can produce to enable you to fight or run. So adrenaline is great stuff, but it has many harmful effects. The heart rate and blood pressure increase, which means more work for the heart. The heart muscle will also require a bigger supply of oxygen. The platelets become sticky and may clump onto the surface of atheromatous plaques in one of your coronary arteries and a heart attack can occur.

Nicotine, by increasing the heart rate and blood pressure,

can increase the frequency and duration of chest pain in those who have angina.

Nicotine can and does increase the excitability of heart muscle, causing extra beats that can lead to serious disturbance in heart rhythm (arrhythmias). Sudden cardiac death is more common in heavy cigarette smokers. The explanation for this is complicated and we will start with a condition you may understand—seizures (epilepsy). In individuals with seizures, the brain cells have a threshold level at which seizures occur. If this threshold is not reached, seizures do not occur. Drugs including alcohol decrease this threshold and seizures are more easily produced, but we can prevent seizures by elevating the threshold. Drugs used to treat epilepsy, for example phenytoin (dilantin), increase the threshold, therefore preventing seizures. Two products of cigarette smoke, nicotine and carbon monoxide, decrease the ventricular fibrillation threshold of heart muscle. The ventricular fibrillation threshold is decreased if the heart muscle is suddenly deprived of blood, or exposed to high concentrations of adrenaline, noradrenaline, and other drugs. During a heart attack, high amounts of noradrenaline are found in and around the damaged muscle and can cause ventricular fibrillation. During ventricular fibrillation the muscle no longer contracts, but quivers. Therefore, the heart is really at a standstill and no blood is being pumped. The heart stops beating, the brain dies; thus there is heart and brain death.

The ventricular fibrillation threshold is slightly increased by only one or two available heart drugs. Beta-blockers counteract the effects of adrenaline and noradrenaline at the cell surface and increase the ventricular fibrillation threshold. I would like to emphasize that since fifty years of research on heart disease have yielded so few useful drugs, we have to salvage every possible assistance from *nondrug* treatment. I hope that this explanation will help you to motivate yourself to stop smoking.

Smokers are inhaling two dangerous compounds, carbon monoxide and nicotine as well as other gases that decrease the ventricular fibrillation threshold and therefore are capable of causing death. This is the one time that you can prevent your death. But we agree, you must be convinced that it is dangerous to smoke so as to be sufficiently motivated to quit. Beware! Lung cancer is common, but heart attacks are very common. There are some of us, the lucky ones, who are immune to all types of knocks including an outpouring of adrenaline, be it from stress, cigarettes, or from other stimuli generated by the body. Therefore, do not use the excuse that your uncle or your aunt or your friends smoke two packs of cigarettes daily and are still living at an age greater than seventy-five. Unfortunately we do not have methods to pick out the 40 or 50 percent of the population that will respond badly to smoking, stress, or a high consumption of saturated fats. Note that hypertension was not listed, as it is a specific disease; we can determine those who have it, and its effects can be documented as well as prevented. Stress, cigarette smoking, and high saturated fat intake are not diseases, and only some individuals exposed to all three factors will develop ill effects. Therefore, it is difficult to talk about prevention unless you understand exactly what is at stake.

It is easy to write and talk about prevention programs, yet it is difficult for many individuals and families to diet and reduce blood cholesterol. Stress is usually inevitable and only a few learn how to live with stress. Discontinuation of smoking, however, only takes the effort of one person. You are the one! Cessation of smoking and the treatment of hypertension are the only two really preventable risk factors. Recognize this, *stop cold turkey*, and save yourself. No one can do it for you. I will outline the other damaging effects of cigarette smoking in an effort to convince you of the danger to your nonsmoking friends, spouse, and children.

## Carbon Monoxide

The hemoglobin of red blood cells transports oxygen to all cells and tissues of the body. Hemoglobin clings to carbon monoxide about 200 times more readily than the oxygen circulating in the blood. In this situation oxygen clings strongly to whatever hemoglobin it can find, and less oxygen is released to the cells. Carbon monoxide combines with hemoglobin to form a compound called carboxyhemoglobin. Therefore, the tissues, including the heart muscle cells, are deprived of oxygen. This is particularly important if the cells are already undernourished and lack oxygen because of severe narrowing of the coronary arteries by atheromatous plaque. These plaques are present in more than 50 percent of North Americans age thirty-five and over. Only about 20 percent are spared from the dreadful atheromatous plaques that cause coronary heart disease. Carboxyhemoglobin likely causes the wall of the arteries to be more permeable to fats including cholesterol, and this can speed up atheroma formation. Individuals with carboxyhemoglobin levels greater than 5 percent are twenty-one times more likely to develop heart attacks or poor circulation in the arteries of the legs than individuals with levels less than 3 percent.[24] There is scientific evidence indicating that heavy cigarette smokers are subjected to eight times the carbon monoxide exposure allowed in industry.[25] You will certainly not stay in a car parked in a closed garage with the engine running knowing the danger of carbon monoxide is death. Do you prefer slow death?

High nicotine or nonnicotine cigarettes produce the same amount of carbon monoxide. Stickiness of the platelets is also increased by carbon monoxide, thus increasing the chance of clotting in the coronary arteries. The ventricular fibrillation threshold of heart muscle and its electrical tissues is reduced by carbon monoxide[26,27]; thus sudden death may not be a mystery. Carbon monoxide is more important than nicotine in causing complications of coronary heart disease, but the two components and many others likely work in concert to orchestrate your departure from this earth.

## SMOKING AND CHEST PAINS

In conditions such as angina, where oxygen supply to the heart muscle is low, the frequency and severity of chest pain may be increased by cigarettes. Nicotine causes a slight increase in blood pressure and heart rate. Therefore, the heart muscle demands more oxygen. Thus, the combination of carbon monoxide and nicotine increases the bad effects. Patients with angina who are smokers develop chest pain at lower levels of exercise.[28]

Other components of cigarette smoking include a glycoprotein that is highly allergenic and may cause shortness of breath, asthmatic attacks, or eye irritation. In addition, the glycoprotein is believed to cause damage to the lining of arteries and an increase in atherosclerosis.

## HABITUATION

This is a major problem because nicotine is a potent chemical that has been conclusively shown to produce addiction and dependence. The smoker will go to extremes to purchase his or her cigarettes and ensure that they are readily available. The craving and hunger can be satisfied by smoking a cigarette or by chewing nicotine-containing gum or by an injection of nicotine.[29] Note that some heavy smokers who stop *cold turkey* do not get symptoms of withdrawal, and you may be one of the lucky.

## IMPOTENCE

Smoking appears to cause a constriction of small penile arteries and may be implicated as one of the many factors responsible for impotence in some individuals.[30]

## EFFECTS ON BYSTANDERS

Inhalation of cigarette smoke by nonsmokers is certainly a concern. The smoke from smoldering cigarettes contains a high concentration of carbon monoxide; smoke exhaled by cigarette smokers in a ventilated or nonventilated room contains enough harmful constituents to cause an increase in heart rate, blood pressure, and carboxyhemoglobin content of the blood of your spouse, children, friends, or bystanders with angina. Therefore it is vital for the public and the various levels of government to insist on nonsmoking areas in all enclosed spaces.

# HOW TO STOP SMOKING

This is a fisherman's story. Everyone who has stopped smoking has his or her own story and will usually try to convince others by telling the awful tale, but with very little effect. I do not pretend to have answers and will not try to give you a plan of how to stop smoking, but will offer a few tips.

Motivation is the key, and this may be achieved by clearly understanding the dangers of cigarette smoking. Nicotine is bad but carbon monoxide is worse. You must bring yourself to believe that cigarette smoking produces enough carbon monoxide to shorten your lifespan. You know that carbon monoxide from motor vehicle exhaust is dangerous and can cause death. It is only a matter of how quickly death will occur. You may knock twenty years off your life if you smoke more than twenty cigarettes daily. Quitting is difficult since nicotine is an addictive chemical. It is best to stop *cold turkey* or reduce to ten cigarettes daily for a few weeks then switch to a low-nicotine brand for two weeks, then stop. Nicotine chewing gum tablets can be helpful at this stage.

It is particularly hard to get teenagers to stop smoking. The emphasis should be to carefully motivate ten- to sixteen-year-olds in schools so that they do not start smoking, or give up the habit of smoking two to ten cigarettes daily since this will soon build up to a larger amount per day. Carefully planned audiovisual programs for class sessions are necessary. These programs must give scientific details including the hazards of the carbon monoxide content of cigarette smoke. I feel that the message regarding carbon monoxide and decrease in ventricular fibrillation threshold is a fruitful area on which to base solid reasoning with the seven- to seventeen-year-old. Audiovisual programs and antismoking literature should incorporate this message. In addition, the video tapes should incorporate the short-term and long-term benefits of not smoking, the incidence of chronic bronchitis, emphysema, lung cancer, and heart attacks. Posters that show a nonsmoking sign with words such as "We urge you not to smoke; beware of the dangers of cigarettes" are not enough to motivate teenagers or seasoned smokers. Nicotine is an addicting drug, and mere words and posters cannot assist the addict. To state that nicotine is addicting seems to carry little weight.

Schools that do not have efficiently run nonsmoking program are certainly not playing their role in the community. School principals should encourage a student body to organize a nonsmoking campaign and should provide the video tape programs. Advice to children is best given by fellow teenagers who are highly motivated and not by teachers or parents. Peer pressure is always effective. The incidence of smoking was reduced in seventh-grade students by using peer role models and active individual role playing.[30] Teenagers are very keen on a ban on nuclear weapons. They are afraid of a nuclear war that would kill millions. The audiovisual programs and circulated leaflets must show that cigarette smoking kills more than a quarter million North Americans yearly, therefore 5 million deaths in twenty years. This is a real-life situation that is as dangerous as a nuclear war that may never occur. Teenagers cannot prevent a nuclear war, but the good news is that teenagers can prevent the deaths of millions by never getting into the habit of smoking.

Parents are very eager to influence their children. The smoking parent by stopping smoking can influence his or her children, especially if they are made aware of the facts outlined in this chapter.

As a bonus, the nonsmoker feels and breathes better and has less difficulty during exercise. At last there is no more dizziness, lightheadedness, mental blocks, or bad breath, which means a better kiss for the teenager. In addition (or as a bonus), the individual drastically reduces the risk of having a fatal or nonfatal heart attack, or chronic bronchitis, emphysema, or lung cancer.

Some techniques to assist with stopping smoking include the following:

1. Participation in stop-smoking clinics and other group programs that emphasize educational and behavioral modification.
2. Nicotine chewing gum or tablets, which are of value and should be tried.
3. Hypnosis, which may be of value to some individuals.

4. Help Health Programs. The American Cancer Society's "I quit kit" with its seven-day program is useful, as well as the National Cancer Institute's "Helping smokers quit kit." (Ask your doctor to obtain a kit for you.) You must develop substitutes; for example, if you feel an urge to smoke, get up, take a walk, talk to someone, or get your favorite book. It is important to engage in an exercise program or at least a half-hour brisk walk twice daily and restrict carbohydrates to prevent weight gain.

*Congratulations, you have quit!* Your smoker's hacking cough will disappear, and your sense of smell and taste will return, and you have added several years to your life.

# CHAPTER 5

# EXERCISE

## BENEFITS OF EXERCISE

One of the main reasons to practice some form of regular, moderate exercise is that it always makes you feel better and look better. Exercise does not have to be vigorous or strenuous to achieve important goals. Important psychological benefits can be produced by moderate exercise such as the combination of walking for twenty minutes, performing stretching exercises for ten minutes, and where possible, cycling or swimming for ten to fifteen minutes daily or at least every second day. These simple exercises are practical, inexpensive, and not time-consuming. In addition, for the individual over age forty, such exercises are of no danger and are sufficient to cause relaxation and produce a sense of well-being and a mental attitude that can better deal with stress.

If you do thirty to forty minutes of moderate exercise a day, and add a favourite sport such as tennis, other racquet sports, or skiing, you will attain a degree of fitness, i.e., you can be considered relatively fit. By "relatively fit," we mean that you have the stamina and energy to do your daily work and favourite sport without shortness of breath, muscle fatigue, or a pounding heart.

Those who seek beyond this achievement are usually age fifteen to forty and approximately 15 percent of the North American population over the age of forty. Individuals who engage in regular vigorous exercise often reach a new "high," and studies have shown that high levels of endorphins are produced in the bodies of such individuals. Endorphins are opiate-like chemicals similar to morphine and these produce an increase in pain threshold and euphoria. With regular vigorous exercise, cardiovascular conditioning is quickly achieved.

It is important to understand some of the terms that are used in describing various types of exercises.

## AEROBIC EXERCISE

Aerobic, isotonic, and dynamic are terms used synony-mously with exercise. Isotonic means "same tension." Aerobic literally means "with air"; i.e., oxygen is required. Isotonic or aerobic exercise involves the rhythmic contraction and relax-ation of large muscle groups and movement of joints, for example, brisk walking, swimming, cycling, jogging, and dancing.

Oxygen is obtained in the lungs and transported by the blood. Your exercising muscles require an increasing supply of oxygen, glucose, and other constituents. The required oxygen is achieved by an increase in the rate of breathing and an increase in heart rate and output of blood from the heart. The amount of blood pumped each minute (cardiac output) increases from the average resting value of about five liters to around twenty liters. A large part of this output goes to the exercising muscles. Aerobic exercises cause an increase in heart rate and an increase in systolic blood pressure; the diastolic blood pressure is unchanged or slightly increased. The blood flow through nonexercising muscles, the liver, intestine, and kidneys, is reduced. If you exercise mainly your upper limbs, this will cause a slightly higher increase in heart rate and blood pressure than exercise utilizing the legs.

## ISOMETRIC, OR STATIC, EXERCISE

Isometric means "equal measure." The muscle fiber length remains the same when muscular tension is exerted against a fixed resistance; i.e., static exercise involves the development

of tension within muscle fibers and results in little or no movement of bones and joints. Weightlifting, pushing against a wall,
or waterskiing are examples. This type of exercise is not
recommended for individuals who are over the age of forty or
who have hypertension or known heart disease since it causes a
marked increase in blood pressure during the effort. The pressure of tensed muscles squeezes blood vessels, and therefore,
less blood passes through these arteries. Also, the constriction
of blood vessels causes an increase in blood pressure. The heart
works harder to pump against the resistance in the constricted
arteries, but the amount of blood the heart pumps only increases slightly since the few muscles that are being used
require less oxygen than would be required during isotonic
exercise. Despite this lower oxygen requirement of the exercising muscle during static exercise, the heart work is increased
and the heart muscle requires more oxygen. If coronary heart
disease is present, the heart muscle may suffer from a shortage
of oxygen that can result in chest pain or angina or precipitation
of a heart attack.

Hypertensive individuals must not engage in static exercises. During static exercise there is an increased heart rate and
blood pressure, but only a mild increase in cardiac output and
rate of breathing. Therefore, physical conditioning may be
achieved but the cardiopulmonary conditioning training effect
cannot be obtained.

## ANAEROBIC EXERCISE

Anaerobic means "without oxygen," and energy is derived
from the breakdown of glucose in the blood and muscle with
the formation of lactic acid. Static exercise such as heavy
weightlifting or very high intensity aerobic exercise such as a
100-yard sprint are examples of anaerobic exercise and heart
patients cannot take part in such exercises.

# CARDIOVASCULAR CONDITIONING— TRAINING EFFECT

When a physically inactive individual suddenly decides to walk up four or five flights of stairs or commences unaccustomed aerobic exercise, he or she quickly gets winded or short of breath and feels the heart thumping away at a fast rate. The lack of physical fitness is obvious to the individual. If the same activity is repeated daily or every other day, after two or three weeks, the individual no longer experiences the shortness of breath; heart rate increases only slightly and there is a faster return to normal resting heart rate after exercise; i.e., the training effect is achieved. Heart, lungs, blood vessels, and muscles have started to adapt.

During exercise, muscles require an increase in oxygen supply. The lungs must take in more oxygen, the heart must pump faster and harder to get the oxygen to the muscles, and the muscles must extract more oxygen.

The heart is a powerful muscular pump but needs oxygen to generate energy for its muscle contraction. The amount of oxygen the heart muscle requires at any point in time (myocardial oxygen consumption) can be determined by complicated techniques. A simple relationship, the product of the heart rate and systolic blood pressure, has been shown to be a reliable indicator of the heart muscle's oxygen requirement. Increased heart muscle efficiency is indicated by a decreased oxygen requirement for a similar amount of work. Regular exercise increases the efficiency of the heart muscle so that it requires less oxygen for the same amount of work. At rest, the heart muscle extracts about 65 percent of the oxygen reaching its muscle cells, and not much more can be extracted on exercise. Therefore if the heart muscle requires more oxygen, the coronary arteries must dilate to supply more oxygenated blood. This situation can occur only if the coronary arteries are normal and capable of dilating.

With frequent exercise the heart becomes conditioned to do the same work at a lower heart rate. You no longer feel your heart pumping away as if it wants to jump out of your chest or throat. If your exercise is then increased both in intensity and duration for at least thirty minutes daily, you will find that your resting heart rate may be reduced by five to twenty beats.

Your heart rate is controlled by the brain and nerves that innervate the heart and the pacemaker (sinus node). The nerves that stimulate the heart to beat faster are called "sympathetic nerves" and they are stimulated from the brain. For example, if someone is going to attack you and you wish to flee, the sympathetic nerves are stimulated by the fright, anxiety, and tension. Noradrenaline produced by the nerve endings and adrenaline by the adrenal glands stimulate the heart to beat faster and stronger.

An opposing nerve called the vagus nerve (parasympathetic nerve) causes the heart to slow down. The "vagus nerve" is like the reins of a horse that keep the horse from running away out of control. Some individuals have an inborn, strong vagal nerve action and have a slow average resting heart rate that is about 64 instead of 72 per minute. Frequent exercise increases the effects of the vagal nerve (tightens the reins) and therefore leads to a slower heart rate. Many athletes have a resting heart rate of 35 to 50 beats per minute so that on exercise the heart rate goes up much less. In an untrained fifty-year-old, a quarter-mile jog may produce a heart rate of 150 to 170 beats per minute. With training, the same exercise may cause a heart rate of only 120 to 140 beats per minute, and the product of heart rate and blood pressure will be reduced. It means that a conditioned heart will not have to work as hard to pump the same amount of blood. The heart muscle therefore requires less oxygen during the exercise.

The coronary arteries fill only when the heart muscle is relaxed (during diastole). A slower heart rate means that the heart is relaxed for a longer period of time and thus has more time to fill the normal or partially obstructed coronary arteries. Therefore, a better supply of oxygen and other nutrients reaches the heart muscle.

A fit heart idles at a lower speed and does not strain during maximal activity; i.e., the difference between the unfit and fit heart is similar to the performance of a poorly tuned 1934 car as opposed to a new 1986 model. However, I must caution that while frequent exercise may slightly lower your heart rate at rest and for a given exercise, all medical experts agree that *there is no scientific evidence that this effect can prevent heart disease of any type*. Importantly, the slower heart rate does not prevent clot formation or atherosclerosis.

During exercise the following important changes occur:

1.  The requirement for oxygen by exercising muscle causes oxygen lack. Therefore the rate at which you breathe increases from about twelve per minute to twenty-four to thirty per minute, so that more oxygen is taken into the lungs and given up to the blood.

2.  Resting muscles extract only about 30 percent of the oxygen from the blood bathing the muscle cells. Vigorously exercising muscle can extract over 75 percent of the circulating oxygen. The amount of oxygen extracted at peak exercise is your maximal oxygen uptake and reflects the limit of your endurance or cardiopulmonary (cardiovascular) conditioning. An increase in your maximal oxygen uptake is the adaptation of the body to aerobic exercise. The body makes more efficient use of the oxygen available and there is also less work for the heart. It is this physiological adaptation that allows you to have more stamina and less fatigue at a given level of aerobic exercise.

## WEIGHT REDUCTION AND EXERCISE

A regular exercise program can cause mild weight reduction, which is greatly enhanced by a weight reduction diet. Exercise is most helpful in long-term weight reduction programs. Physical activity requires energy, which is measured in calories. Think of the body as having several factories. If you shut down half of these factories and let the other half work at half the speed, your output would be diminished. This is equivalent to turning down your metabolic rate (metabolic thermostat). If you go on a crash diet, your metabolic thermostat is turned down to get by on less food. Twenty to forty minutes of aerobic exercise done regularly three to four times weekly can boost your metabolic rate by 20 to 30 percent, and this will accelerate breakdown of fat stores. The body of an obese individual is programmed to form fat and to store it away. In addition, your cells slow down and you burn fewer calories than normal. Cells slow down even more if you are on a severe weight reduction diet so as to conserve energy. The more you exercise, the more dependent you become on fat metabolism. Many obese individuals do not overeat, but their metabolic rate is so low that they store fat. Therefore, start your exercise first, then a few weeks later start your weight reduction diet and continue on an exercise program for at least one year to keep the weight down.

To burn 100 calories, a 170-pound individual needs to walk briskly 1½ miles or jog one mile. Note that brisk walking is nearly as good as jogging since the speed at which you complete the distance makes little difference to the total amount of calories you burn. Therefore, a brisk mile in 15 minutes twice daily or two miles once daily is of value until you can add other exercises. If you do this daily, you will loose one pound in less than fourteen days. If your diet usually provides 1,200 to 1,500 calories daily and you drop to a 1,000-calorie diet during this exercise program, you will have an additional one-pound loss in fourteen days. This may seem small, but the good news is that in six months you will be twenty-four pounds lighter and you will be able to hold on to this reduction. Now that you are used to exercise, if you continue your program four days weekly, you will find it is easy to stay on a 1,000- to 1,200-calorie diet and you will maintain ideal weight. Exercise alone without restriction of calorie intake results in only mild weight reduction. Therefore, both exercise and diet should be used to achieve the best results.

## EFFECTS ON BLOOD PRESSURE

Blood pressure is not significantly lowered during vigorous exercise. I must emphasize that during vigorous exercise such as five miles of jogging or twenty minutes of continuous aerobic exercise, the systolic blood pressure increases markedly in most individuals. In many, the rise in blood pressure is substantial and it is possible that damage can occur in arteries during the months of vigorous exercise. For example, a thirty-year-old with a normal systolic blood pressure of 120 mm Hg, on running one to two miles, will usually have an increase in blood pressure during the run to about 140 to 180; there is usually no increase in the diastolic blood pressure except in patients who have hypertension. Blood pressure rapidly falls on cessation of exercise and returns to the normal resting level within a few minutes. Individuals with mild hypertension who engage in a regular exercise program may obtain a mild reduction in their resting blood pressure and this is believed to be due to a combination of factors including weight loss and relaxation. Therefore, indirectly, regular exercises are important to assist with weight reduction, thereby lowering blood pressure in individuals with mild hypertension. If you have moderate or severe hypertension, do not depend on exercise; it will not reduce blood pressure and can cause an increase in existing high blood pressure during vigorous exercise. We cannot exclude the possibility that damage to arteries may be increased by vigorous exercise in some individuals.

## EFFECTS ON THE BLOOD

Regular vigorous exercise increases high-density lipoprotein ("good") cholesterol from 1 to 15 percent. It is debatable whether this slight rise in HDL cholesterol decreases risk over a long period of time. Moderate exercise has a variable effect. The total blood cholesterol and low-density lipoprotein ("bad") cholesterol are not significantly reduced by exercise. Elevated triglycerides are reduced by exercise, but elevated triglycerides are not considered to be a risk factor for coronary heart disease.

Other effects of vigorous exercise include a variable effect on blood-clotting factors. A substance in the blood, factor VIII, is necessary for blood clotting and is absent in bleeders (hemophiliacs). Hemophiliacs who exercise get a mild and helpful increase in factor VIII. Vigorous exercise in healthy individuals increases factor VIII, as well as the number and stickiness of platelets. This is offset in healthy young individuals by a mild increase in factors that tend to dissolve blood clots. Importantly, in individuals over age fifty, or at any age if atherosclerosis of the artery is present, the ability to dissolve clots is impaired. Consequently, small clots (thrombi) may form on plaques of atheroma, thus increasing their size; and slowly, over five to ten years, this may cause or promote existing coronary heart disease. Walking at a rate of four miles per hour, however, does not cause an increase in factor VIII or platelets, and the stickiness of platelets is slightly reduced. Therefore, "Walk and win! Miles for millions."

## DOES EXERCISE PREVENT FATAL OR NONFATAL HEART ATTACKS?

The exercise craze is in vogue, and millions of North Americans participate in regular exercise programs. This is a major achievement motivated by various advertisements and literature and the desire to feel fit as well as possibly to stay alive longer. Only time and further research studies will answer the question regarding exercise and longevity.

A few studies have suggested that cardiac death is more common in sedentary individuals than in the physically active. But further analysis of these studies revealed major defects in methodology and interpretation. Published studies on exercise and the risk of coronary heart disease lack standardization of the diagnosis of coronary heart disease, information on the effects of associated risk factors, and reliable evaluation of recreational or occupational physical activity.

Studies include the following:

1. To assess the role of physical exertion in relation to risk of fatal heart attack, the 1951–1972 work experience of 6,351 San Francisco longshoremen was studied.[32] Among men age 35 to 54 there were 24 heart attack deaths in those engaged in heavy work, 37 deaths in men classified as doing moderate work and 28 deaths in those engaged in light work. Thus, there was no difference in the death rates in men age 35 to 54. Among men age 65 to 74 there were 8 deaths in men

engaged in heavy work six months prior to death, 9 deaths in those engaged in moderate work and 275 deaths in those engaged in light work six months before death. Each man who had a fatal heart attack was classified in the job category that he held six months before death. This study is controversial because of errors in methodology. Men 64 plus are usually engaged in light work activity and death is expected in this age group. We know that the 275 men, age over 64, who died were engaged in light work six months prior to death but the study does not indicate what their activity level was during age 35 to 64.

2. A study done in 1966 showed that London bus drivers had a slightly higher incidence of heart attacks than London bus conductors, but other risk factors confounded the analysis.[33] For example, from the outset, the bus drivers were heavier, with a higher blood pressure and blood cholesterol than bus conductors and were, therefore, at higher risk. These risk factors were probably more important than job activity classification.

3. In the seven-country collaborative study, moderately active Finns had a 2½ times higher incidence of coronary heart disease than the least active and the most active Finns.[7] Confounding factors in this study included a high incidence of elevated blood cholesterol, which may have modified the effects of increased physical activity.

4. In a study of 17,000 male university alumni, 2,000 kilocalories (kcal) of exercise per week slightly reduced the risk of coronary heart disease.[34] Vigorous sports, climbing stairs, and walking to obtain a minimum of 500 kcal of exercise per week appeared to be necessary to obtain a reduced coronary artery disease risk.

5. An Australian study utilized 370 men who took part in a twice weekly exercise program with one hour of calisthenics, volleyball, and running so as to improve physical fitness by 17 percent.[35] The program was continued for five years, and even though the men felt physically fit, there was no reduction in blood cholesterol, weight, or blood pressure. Other studies sup-

port the view that moderate exercise does not significantly alter "risk factors" for coronary heart disease.

6. Morris et al. analysed the exercise habits of 18,000 sedentary male office workers.[36] Those with vigorous leisure time activity had about a 50 percent reduction in heart attacks. The 1,800 men were asked on a Monday morning to complete a record indicating their level of physical activity on the preceding Friday and Saturday. In this study, vigorous exercise included (a) sports and recreation, i.e., singles tennis, swimming, jogging, running, walking at a rate of four miles per hour, cycling fast uphill; and (b) very heavy work. At the end of 8½ years, there were 24 (1.1%) fatal and 42 (2%) nonfatal heart attacks in the vigorous-exercise group of 2,200 men, but 411 (2.9%) fatal and 570 (4%) nonfatal heart attacks in the nonvigorous-exercise group of 16,800 men. Thus there was about a 50 percent reduction in heart attacks attributed to the good effects of vigorous exercise. These results are statistically significant. However, selection of individuals may have created a bias and the study can be criticized.

7. Marathon running does not offer any guarantees and it is not believed to be as protective as some enthusiasts would have us believe.[37] In four of seven marathoners who had completed a total of sixty-four marathons and died, autopsy showed severe atherosclerosis of their coronary arteries. The bad news is that severe coronary atherosclerosis is the commonest cause of death, even among marathoners.

It is worth noting that in Finland there is a high occupational level of physical exertion, yet coronary heart disease mortality is very high.

The public must understand that exercise has important benefits *but it cannot be expected to halt the progression or complications of coronary heart disease*. Exercise enthusiasts must recognize that control of other risk factors and prevention of clotting are more important than exercise in preventing heart attacks.

# RISKS OF EXERCISE AND PRECIPITATION OF HEART ATTACKS, SUDDEN DEATH, OR HEART FAILURE

The relationship between vigorous exercise and the risk of a fatal or nonfatal heart attack has long been the subject of controversy. A study reported in the *New England Journal of Medicine*, October 1984, showed that vigorous exercise can precipitate sudden cardiac death in healthy individuals.[38] The risk of sudden death is higher in men with low levels of habitual activity who engage in unusual vigorous exercise. However, even in men who were accustomed to vigorous activity, the risk of sudden cardiac death was moderately increased during high-intensity exercise. This study did create a stir.

However, I must emphasize that the authors only analyzed nine deaths. It would be foolhardy to make any generalizations from such a study. The study was done in King County, Washington, an area containing 1.25 million people. Only nine cardiac arrests during vigorous exercise occurred in fourteen months—five in men with low levels of habitual activity and four in men with high levels of activity. This study should not influence the medical profession or public except to emphasize that jogging is relatively safe and cardiac arrest is very rare. However, sedentary individuals must take heed not to rush out and do vigorous exercises without engaging in levels of gradual activity. In addition, in Rhode Island during a six-year period, only one jogging death occurred per year for every 6,720 joggers.[39] This is a very low death rate but is higher than expected. Despite my defense of jogging for those who love it, I must emphasize that all studies show a much higher incidence of heart attacks during exercise than would be expected by chance. Heart attack is the commonest cause of death during exercise.[38-41]

The death of exercise enthusiast James Fixx is a good example of nonprotection by exercise. In his early thirties he recognized that he was at high risk since his family history was strong for heart attacks before age fifty. A daily run of five to ten miles for more than fifteen years did not protect him from the silent killer.

Note that during jogging and running, the systolic blood pressure may be slightly or moderately increased. The combined increase in blood pressure and high-velocity blood flow may over a period of years increase atherosclerosis.

Strenuous exercise can precipitate death in individuals who have a very rare heart muscle problem called obstructive cardiomyopathy. The division (septum) between the right and left ventricle becomes extremely thick for reasons unknown and it obstructs the blood flow from the left ventricle into the aorta. This condition explains the rare sudden death that occurs in some athletes under the age of thirty. This obstructive heart muscle problem is fortunately very rare and is easy to exclude by a doctor listening with a stethoscope and with added tests such as an ECG and an echocardiogram (ultrasound of the heart).

All patients with known heart disease or with symptoms that suggest heart disease—pain or discomfort in the chest, throat, jaw, or arms during activity; shortness of breath; palpitations (fast, pounding heartbeats or skipped heartbeats)—should have an assessment by a doctor and a stress test before engaging in moderate or vigorous exercise. Patients with previous heart failure or marked heart enlargement should engage only in moderate exercise such as walking or its equivalent. Exercise is well known to precipitate heart failure in such individuals and therefore further advice from your doctor is necessary if you want to do exercise other than the equivalent of walking one mile.

## INJURIES DURING JOGGING

The up and down motion of jogging often causes tendon, muscle, and joint injuries. In one survey, about 1,800 injuries occurred in 1,650 amateur runners. Injuries included: (1) Achilles' tendinitis: the heel and tendon become painful; (2) shin splints: the muscles at the front of the leg (frontal compartment syndrome) become painful and swollen; (3) painful knees: inflammation of the fluid-filled sac (bursitis), strain on ligaments, or painful knee caps (chondromalacia patellae); (4) painful feet:

inflammation of the sole of the foot, plantar fasciitis, and trauma to the bones of the foot; and (5) exacerbation of arthritis of the hips, knees, and ankles. Patients with arthritis must not jog. Women are more susceptible to knee injuries or stress fractures in the pelvis, and in some, osteoporosis (loss of bone) may develop.

If you must jog, purchase good running shoes, exercise the ankle joint, and warm up properly to prevent injuries. Despite such maneuvers, injuries are very common among joggers.

## HOW TO START AN EXERCISE PROGRAM

If you are under thirty-five, do not have arthritis or moderate or severe hypertension, and feel in good health, you can engage in all activities including vigorous exercise as frequently as you desire. Regardless of age, it is wise to do five to ten minutes warm-up exercises before going on to vigorous exercises. Warm-up exercises prevent the pulse and blood pressure from increasing abruptly, thereby putting sudden strain on the heart. You should engage for one to two weeks in moderate exercise such as walking one to two miles, or jogging one mile daily before considering vigorous aerobic exercise such as running two to five miles three or four times weekly. If you are under thirty-five, there is very little reason to check the pulse rate. If you feel your heart pounding away very rapidly, then slow your pace. For those engaged in competitive sports: I am in agreement with other experts, that running is perhaps the best exercise for those who require the stamina to do the utmost. The swimmer, boxer, or cyclist should jog and run to develop stamina and strengthen other muscles. Similarly, the runner should engage in other exercises, especially swimming and cycling.

*For individuals over age thirty-five* in good health, the following advice is given:

1.  Walking two miles in a half hour, swimming, or cycling are excellent exercises. They are efficient and safe, as well as economical. Walking four miles in an

hour and climbing six flights of stairs daily can produce cardiovascular conditioning. You do not require special equipment and you do not have to travel to a gym or ski slope or racquet club. Walking two miles quickly burns up as many calories as jogging one mile. Jogging exercises the legs, but not the important quadriceps muscles at the front of the thighs. Walking up three to six flights of stairs daily or cycling will strengthen the quadriceps; strong quadriceps strengthen and stabilize the knees.

2. If you are physically inactive at work and at home for more than six months, you should start very slowly. Start with daily or alternate-day ten-minute stretching exercises, moving all the joints and the muscles of the upper and lower limbs as well as the trunk. Follow with twenty minutes of brisk walking (a little more than a mile), and then cycle for five to ten minutes. A stationary bicycle is a good investment. After about four weeks of this mild exercise, increase the walk to thirty minutes and cycle for ten to fifteen minutes. After one month of this routine, if you feel well with no abnormal symptoms such as chest, throat, or arm discomfort, very fast heartbeats or shortness of breath, you can freely engage in your favorite racquet sport. Swimming is well known to be an excellent conditioner as well as pleasurable exercise. If you wish to move to vigorous exercise, you should have a medical checkup. It is a pity that many individuals commence jogging or other exercise at twenty-eight and stop at thirty-five. For some it is a pleasure and for others an obsession that imposes stress. Those who love jogging should obviously continue, especially through the vulnerable years—ages thirty-five to fifty-five.

## HEART RATE: MAXIMUM AND TRAINING RANGE

Learn to take your heart rate and determine your maximal and submaximal heart rate. During your medical checkup, your doctor will show you how to feel the pulse at the wrist (radial artery) or the carotid artery in the neck. Count the pulse beat for ten seconds and multiply the number by six to get the heart rate per minute.

The heart rate increases to high levels with vigorous exercise and these upper limits have been established by doctors engaged in exercise conditioning programs.

Several charts have been designed by experts and used in different countries. At age twenty the highest heart rate that the normal heart can achieve is between 200 and 220 beats per minute, and this is called the maximum attainable heart rate (Table 5-1). To be safe, doctors advise that you should not exceed 85 percent of this maximal value, that is, about 170 per minute if you are young, and healthy. During the first few weeks of training, keep the heart rate at about 70 percent maximum, that is, about 140 beats per minute, and increase the exercise to get to 85 percent if you are under age 30. If you are in good health, it is safe to exercise so that your heart rate reaches 70 to 85 percent of your maximal and to keep it at this rate for about twenty minutes. After six to eight weeks of strenuous exercise, you should achieve physical and cardiopulmonary conditioning. At age forty your maximum heart rate should be approximately 220 − 40, or 180, and your training range—your "target zone"—from 125 to 150; i.e., your pulse counted for ten seconds should be a minimum of twenty and a maximum of twenty-five beats. However, I must emphasize, that you do not necessarily need to reach and maintain the target zone, as some have claimed, to obtain conditioning—the training effect.

## TABLE 5-1 AGE-RELATED MAXIMUM ATTAINABLE HEART RATES AND TRAINING RANGE

| Age | | 20 | 25 | 30 | 35 | 40 | 45 | 50 | 55 | 60 | 65 |
|---|---|---|---|---|---|---|---|---|---|---|---|
| Maximum Heart Rate (220 − age) | | 200 | 195 | 190 | 185 | 180 | 175 | 170 | 165 | 160 | 155 |
| Training Zone | 85% | 170 | 165 | 161 | 157 | 153 | 148 | 145 | 140 | 135 | 130 |
| | 70% | 140 | 136 | 133 | 130 | 126 | 122 | 120 | 115 | 112 | 108 |

Maximum rates and training ranges are given in Table 5-1. Individuals over age forty who have not engaged in strenuous exercise in the last two years or who have a family history of heart attacks before age fifty, or blood cholesterol greater than 220 mg, or mild hypertension—are advised to have a stress test before starting vigorous exercise.

## STRESS TEST

A stress test involves walking on the treadmill or cycling while your ECG is being continuously recorded. The ECG terminals are taped onto your chest. Walking on the treadmill is easier if you wear running shoes or other comfortable flat shoes. The treadmill speed and its inclination are programmed to increase every three minutes so that you walk faster up a grade and are jogging by the tenth minute. Healthy individuals are exercised to 90 percent of their maximal heart rate. The test is discontinued if chest or leg pain, fatigue, or shortness of breath develops or if the electrocardiogram shows insufficient oxygen to the heart muscle. The blood pressure is taken every three minutes and the systolic blood pressure usually rises by 20 to 40 mm Hg. A forty-year-old who is physically fit with good cardiopulmonary condition can usually exercise for ten to twelve minutes, reaching a heart rate of 160 to 170 beats per minute without having undue shortness of breath. The test is completed by a few minutes of slow walking to cool down before the treadmill is turned off.

A well-conditioned thirty-five-year-old athlete's heart rate may increase only to 120 to 140 per minute during twelve minutes of such exercise; on resting, the heart rate should fall quickly to under 100 per minute within one to four minutes. The same cool-down period should apply in your exercise at home. When you have completed your vigorous exercise, always cool down for two to five minutes by walking around, doing some stretching, or going up and down stairs a few times.

Exercise prescriptions for patients who have heart disease, especially coronary heart disease, are discussed in Chapter 10, "How to Deal with Heart Attacks."

# CONCLUSION

I strongly recommend regular, moderate exercise for healthy individuals and those with coronary heart disease. Fitness makes one feel like living and confers a sense of well-being. If you are relatively fit, you can enjoy your favorite sport with better breathing capabilities and without feeling your heart pounding. If you are fit, you are not likely to be overweight, your clothes fit you better, and you feel better and look better. I strongly recommend regular moderate exercise to achieve a state of "relative fitness."

I recommend vigorous exercise to those who are young, healthy, and already fit. A fit heart idles at a slower speed. A heart that beats slower allows better filling of normal or partially obstructed coronary arteries. However, at present, there is no scientific proof or adequate evidence to suggest that vigorous exercise will make you live longer.[42] If you are over age forty, mainly sedentary, and engage in occasional mild exercise, do not start vigorous exercise without having a medical check or stress test. Start with walking one to two miles daily, slowly adding cycling, swimming, or similar exercise. Avoid vigorous exercise until you have done more than three months of daily moderate exercise.

Vigorous exercise in previously inactive individuals over age thirty-five carries a high risk of fatal or nonfatal heart attacks or sudden death.[38] Therefore, do not rush to get superfit. Get fit slowly over three to six months, remembering that fitness is a relative term—fit to do what?

In addition, I emphasize that simple exercises—walking two miles in a half hour or when possible four miles in an hour, climbing stairs, or peddling a stationary bicycle for 15 minutes—are excellent safe exercises. Walking is always helpful and "never" causes a heart attack. It does not increase blood pressure; it improves circulation in the legs and may have a favorable influence on blood clotting. Therefore if you walk, you may win the *race*!

# CHAPTER 6

# STRESS

Stress is not really nervous tension, so I will not dwell on the subject of nervousness and chronic anxiety, the cause of which must be determined and removed. Damaging or unpleasant stress, as Hans Selye states, is "stress with distress and this is always disagreeable."[43] Although stress can be associated with pleasant situations, it is more often produced in the individual by unpleasant stimuli. The word "stress" is derived from the Old French and Middle English words for "distress," and although the first syllable was lost over the years, it is best to use the word "stress" only when there is distress.

There is no doubt that stress is awful. With the exception of severe pain and death, severe stress with distress is one of the most difficult situations we have to face. Stress is nearly always present at work; it is a part of living. However, if stress is accompanied by distress, there is harm.

Stress produces well-known reactions in the body, in particular, an increase in blood pressure, and causes small blood particles (platelets) to become sticky. The platelet particles stick together to form clumps or sludge, which can lead to formation of a blood clot in the coronary artery.

Trauma to your arteries reeks havoc like a silent curse, a silent killer. During the stress reaction, the arteries constrict under the influence of adrenaline; consequently both systolic and diastolic blood pressure increase. If your blood pressure is usually 120/80, it can go up to 160/90, or from 145/95 to as high as 190/110. These elevated pressures, lasting only minutes, are injurious to the arteries, and when combined with the effects of

66

excess adrenaline, causing platelet sludging in the arteries, we see the death toll from heart attacks rising.

How does stress cause heart pain (angina) and damage to the heart and arteries? When the coronary arteries are narrowed by plaques of atheroma, chest pain may occur (Figures 1-1 and 1-4). Chest pain is made worse by exertion such as walking up a hill. However, pain at rest may occur if the patient faces sudden emotional upset. The individual may feel a distress in the chest.

Stress causes adrenaline and noradrenaline release. These stress hormones cause the heart rate and blood pressure to increase, giving the heart more work to do (Figure 6-1). Adrenaline and noradrenaline have similar effects and the terms are interchangeable. In some patients, adrenaline may cause platelets to clump onto plaques of atheroma, thus causing oxygen lack to that segment of heart muscle. This oxygen lack may or may not produce chest pain.

Moderate stress associated with simple daily activities can decrease the blood supply to the heart muscle in patients with coronary heart disease. In a study of sixteen patients who had angina, the moderate stress of mental arithmetic caused oxygen lack to the heart muscle (myocardial ischemia) similar to that produced by exercise.[44] In these patients a radioisotope material (rubidium-82) was injected into a vein, and when it reached the heart muscle, photographs were taken. The dark areas in Figure 6-2 represent the uptake of blood supply to the heart muscle. When the supply of blood is decreased, the area of muscle is poorly supplied with blood, the presence of the radioisotope, rubidium-82, is reduced, and the area of darkness is diminished. The simple stress of mental arithmetic causes lack of blood to the heart muscle.

In a similar experiment, a patient who was having catheterization of his heart (coronary arteriogram) was asked to do mental arithmetic, was asked to think of a past stressful situation, and was shown the result of his catheter studies. His heart muscle function was determined during the test and showed no significant change with thinking of past stress, but showed a mild defect during mental arithmetic and severe defects in muscle function during the explanation and viewing of the findings of his heart catheter test.[45]

A stressful situation causes the "emotional center" in the

## Figure 6-1. Stress And The Heart

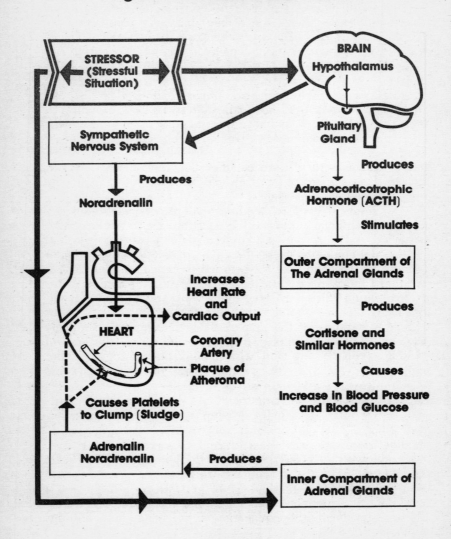

# Figure 6-2. The Heart Under Stress

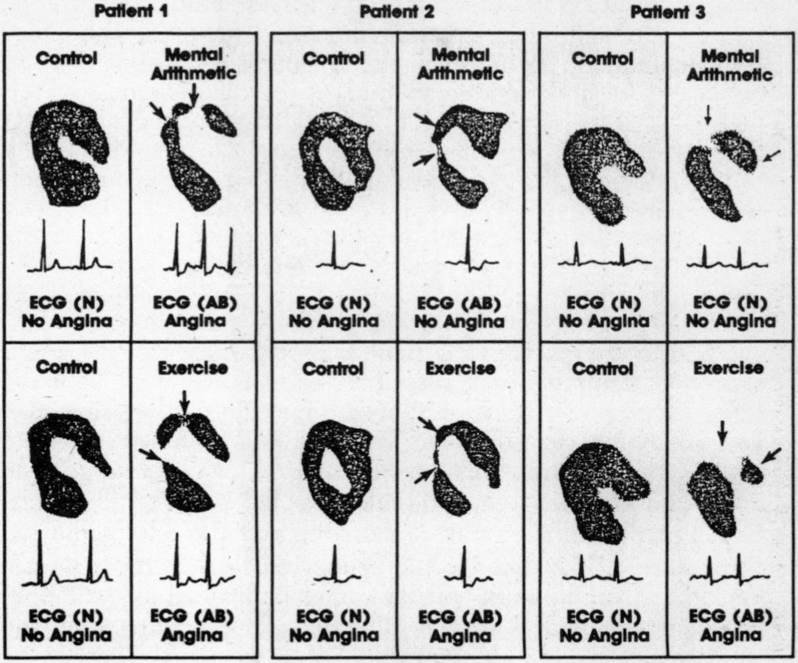

Changes in the uptake of rubidium-82 and the electro-cardiogram in relation to chest pain before and after mental arithmetic or exercise.

Control scans, dark areas, show normal rubidium-82 uptake by the heart muscle in three patients, indicating normal blood flow.

There are defects in uptake (arrows) with mental arithmetic and exercise, and these changes can be accompanied by ECG changes of oxygen lack to the muscle= ischemia=angina.

**N = Normal    AB = Abnormal**

Modified from Lancet 2: 1003, 1984 (with permission)

brain to trigger certain reactions (Figure 6-1). The hypothalamus sends signals to the pituitary gland and sympathetic nervous system, which leads to secretion of "stress hormones," cortisone, adrenaline, and noradrenaline. Cortisone causes an increase in blood glucose and an increase in blood pressure.

As a result of a stressful situation (stressor), the inner compartment of the adrenal glands pours out adrenaline and noradrenaline and these compounds are involved in the "fight or flight" reaction.

The external stimulus (stressor) is usually a condition that produces anger, fear, anxiety, deprivation, and the like. Common stressors include the death of a spouse, conflicts with others, projects requiring a deadline. Very often the stressor consists of "words" that are interpreted by the individual as harsh or hurtful, resulting in anger, hostility, humiliation, or resentment.

The body reacts in the same way regardless of the type or source of stress or unexpressed anger. An argument with the boss, fellow workers, your spouse, or others is the same as if you are being chased by an assailant. The fight for so-called prestige, recognition, and survival at work or at home goes on daily, and for many years you may bear the brunt of the attack. You are riled to the point of bursting and the adrenaline has been poured. Visualize the adrenaline as little death potions that one may drink at work and for some, unfortunately, at home. Adrenaline is helpful in some situations; for example, when you want to flee from a charging bull or an assailant. These compounds increase the heart rate and blood pressure and increase the supply of blood containing glucose and oxygen to exercising muscles so that you are able to run. However, too much adrenaline, and in particular noradrenaline, can be dangerous since these chemicals can overstimulate the heart, disturb its electrical stability, and on rare occasions, lead to ventricular fibrillation, during which the heart does not contract but quivers. This condition is the usual cause of sudden death. Noradrenaline and adrenaline cause a decrease in the ventricular fibrillation threshold, which means that the heart quivers more quickly. Adrenaline causes platelets to clump, and if this occurs on a plaque of atheroma, pain can occur or a clot can develop. These compounds can also cause spasm of the coronary arteries, which in turn can produce chest pain and sometimes death, especially if the spasm occurs where the plaque partially blocks the artery.

As outlined earlier, heart deaths are due to two major problems:

1. Formation of a blood clot in the coronary artery.
2. Electrical disturbances that cause the heart to quiver and not contract (ventricular fibrillation).

Sudden death is common, and the possibility cannot be excluded that severe acute stress may cause death by initiating a brain-adrenaline-heart interaction (Figure 6-1). The clumping of platelets can enlarge the plaque, and over a period of years, the buildup of clot on a plaque can cause complete obstruction of the arteries, therefore, a heart attack. Animal experiments lend support to this hypothesis. Rats exposed to sudden trauma such as being plunged into ice water develop blockage of the coronary arteries, which results in damage to the segments of the heart muscle (myocardial infarction). When rats were not physically traumatized, but were stressed with nonphysically traumatic electric shocks, they developed clots in the coronary arteries and died.[46] When rats were pretreated with drugs that prevent platelet clumping, such as aspirin or dipyridamole, and then subjected to similar electric shocks, clots were prevented in the majority.[46, 47]

Experimentally, adrenaline or noradrenaline given intravenously can cause severe electrical disturbances and the heart just quivers. During a heart attack, there is an increase in noradrenaline in the heart muscle. When blood flow to the heart is reduced by atherosclerosis of the coronary artery, severe stress can more easily precipitate ventricular fibrillation. There are several reports in the scientific literature that document these occurrences. I have personally observed such cases. For example: A male, age fifty-eight, had a heart attack and was quite well for the next year. While watching his son play hockey, he had a cardiac arrest due to ventricular fibrillation, but was successfully resuscitated. He did well for about ten months and during that time avoided hockey games in which his son played. One unfortunate day he ventured out to see his son play; during the excitement of the hockey game, he had a sudden cardiac arrest with ventricular fibrillation and died.

When a coronary artery is suddenly blocked in dogs, severe quivering of the heart occurs in some. However, when the hypothalamus (in the brain) and sympathetic nervous system are stimulated to produce noradrenaline at the same time that the coronary artery is blocked, quivering of the heart frequently occurs.[48] Beta-blocking drugs block the actions of adrenaline and noradrenaline, and if dogs are pretreated with these drugs and the coronary artery is then blocked, the dangerous quivering of the heart can be prevented.[49]

In a study involving 117 patients who were resuscitated from cardiac arrest, 25 reported that they had severe stress such as job and family conflicts within the twenty-four hours prior to the cardiac arrest.[50] Acute or prolonged (chronic) stress may produce severe damage to the coronary arteries. You must remember that atheroma of the arteries commonly produces no symptoms; it is a silent killer. After many years, a clot develops on an atheromatous plaque. There is considerable evidence linking increased stickiness of platelets to the production of atheroma.

## STRESS AND SPORTS

Do not push yourself to jog or run. Do it if you feel great and happy without having to clench your jaws or tighten your facial muscles. If you have to push yourself to do an additional mile, then you may secrete excess adrenaline and noradrenaline and this takes its toll on your cardiovascular system throughout the years. Similarly, be careful not to be overly competitive when playing racquet sports. No one gets hurt under age thirty, but if you are more than forty, very competitive vigorous sports such as squash and racquetball can occasionally hurt your cardiovascular system.

# THE SYMPTOMS AND SIGNS OF STRESS

1.  You immediately feel sweaty, especially on the forehead, on the skull, under the armpits, and on the palms owing to the presence of excess adrenaline.
2.  Your heart races and may easily pound.
3.  An ache in the head and neck especially in your temples or eyes.
4.  A feeling of turmoil, or tightness in the chest or stomach. You may feel as if there were butterflies in your stomach, or there is a feeling of anguish, terror, fright, restlessness, agitation, or tremulousness. You may feel shaky, jittery, or weak all over.
5.  Speech is slurred and you feel that you cannot even scream or talk for a few seconds.
6.  You may feel hostile, violent, full of rage and anger, and ready to fight back.
7.  You have difficulty sleeping.
8.  You may experience frequency of urination, indigestion, or sometimes diarrhea.

# HOW TO HANDLE STRESS

Stress is a part of living and cannot be completely avoided. When you understand how traumatic stress can be to your heart and arteries, you may be motivated to develop techniques to deal with stress.

Stress management is a complex subject, beyond the scope of this book. Therefore, I will not attempt to give specific stress management techniques.

Some of the ways that are indicated to cope with stress include mental diversion, techniques to develop a healthy self-concept, time management, progressive deep relaxation techniques, meditation, biofeedback, and exercise.

## CONCLUSION

I believe that stress is as important as the major "risk factors," but it is difficult to prove this hypothesis scientifically. Stress, cholesterol, hypertension, smoking, and blood-clotting factors work in concert in the genetically susceptible individual to produce atherosclerosis and, finally, a fatal or nonfatal heart attack. A stressor causes the sympathetic nervous system and adrenal glands to secrete stress hormones, which increase the work of the heart, and cause platelet clumping that can sometimes cause a blood clot in the coronary artery. I have outlined how excess adrenaline and noradrenaline alter the electrical stability of the heart, predisposing it to a high risk of a curious quivering (ventricular fibrillation) during which it fails to contract, and sudden death may occur.

Human beings are fortunate that the working of the body is such that the reaction caused by one chemical is often counterbalanced by other chemicals that are produced in the body. Nature does not always win, but it can, with a little help from a friend—you! I strongly urge you to develop strategies that may enable you to deal with various stressful situations. Thus you will be able to handle stress and *subdue the brain-adrenaline-heart-artery-reaction,* described above.

---

# CHAPTER 7

# ROLE OF OBESITY, DIABETES, TRIGLYCERIDES, ALCOHOL, VITAMINS, ESTROGEN HORMONES, AND TYPE A BEHAVIOR

## OBESITY

If you are slightly or moderately overweight, this does not increase your risk of having a heart attack, provided that you do not have other risk factors—especially hypertension, hypercholesterolemia (high blood cholesterol), smoking, and diabetes. The notion that being overweight is detrimental to health has been in vogue for many years. The news media and those interested in prescribing their new weight loss diets have portrayed the issue as if it were a scientific fact. A renowned scientific expert is adamant that the idea has been greatly exploited and that there is no increased risk if you are middle-aged and moderately overweight.[51]

The 1983 Metropolitan height and weight tables are given in Table 7–1. If you are slightly overweight, you would be happy to learn that the earlier Metropolitan Life tables of ideal or average weights were derived from insurance applicants age twenty to thirty and do not represent the average weights of individuals age forty to sixty. If your weight is 10 percent more than that indicated in Table 7–1, you can consider yourself slightly overweight, but there is still no health hazard unless you have other risk factors. The average weight of North Americans age thirty to fifty is about 10 to 15 percent above those indicated in Table 7-1. Many North Americans age thirty-five to sixty-five are overweight, even by the conservative definition given above. If you are in this group and have other risk factors, you need to reduce your weight. The Framingham Study showed that in the 5,000 residents, being overweight appeared to increase the risk of sudden death and angina, but it did not increase the frequency of heart attacks.[52] When adjustments were made for the prevalance of hypertension and hypercholesterolemia, then overweight or obesity appeared to play a much less significant role. If a patient with chest pain due to coronary heart disease is overweight, chest pains are likely to be more frequent, as the heart certainly has more work to do. Therefore, weight reduction does help in relieving pain in patients with angina pectoris, and it is advisable.

TABLE 7–1
1983 METROPOLITAN HEIGHT AND WEIGHT TABLES FOR
MEN AND WOMEN
According to Frame, Ages 25–59

|  | MEN | | |
| HEIGHT (In Shoes)† Feet Inches | Weight in Pounds (In Indoor Clothing)* | | |
| | SMALL FRAME | MEDIUM FRAME | LARGE FRAME |
|---|---|---|---|
| 5   2 | 128–134 | 131–141 | 138–150 |
| 5   3 | 130–136 | 133–143 | 140–153 |
| 5   4 | 132–138 | 135–145 | 142–156 |
| 5   5 | 134–140 | 137–148 | 144–160 |
| 5   6 | 136–142 | 139–151 | 146–164 |
| 5   7 | 138–145 | 142–154 | 149–168 |
| 5   8 | 140–148 | 145–157 | 152–172 |
| 5   9 | 142–151 | 148–160 | 155–176 |
| 5   10 | 144–154 | 151–163 | 158–180 |
| 5   11 | 146–157 | 154–166 | 161–184 |
| 6   0 | 149–160 | 157–170 | 164–188 |
| 6   1 | 152–164 | 160–174 | 168–192 |
| 6   2 | 155–168 | 164–178 | 172–197 |
| 6   3 | 158–172 | 167–182 | 176–202 |
| 6   4 | 162–176 | 171–187 | 181–207 |

* Indoor clothing weighing 5 pounds for men and 3 pounds for women.
† Shoes with 1-inch heels.

You are considered obese if you are more than 25 percent above the average weight and have a high percentage of body fat. You are moderately obese if you are 25 to 50 percent above the average weight and have marked increase in body fat. Measurement of body mass index, from your weight divided by the square of your height, is a useful measure of relative obesity.[53]

Obesity is not a major cause of hypertension, but some obese patients do have an increase in blood pressure. If you are obese and lose weight, the blood pressure always falls. A significant number of obese patients have diabetes and elevated blood cholesterol, and if hypertension or cigarette smoking are added, the risk is considerably increased.

TABLE 7–1
1983 METROPOLITAN HEIGHT AND WEIGHT TABLES FOR MEN AND WOMEN
According to Frame, Ages 25–59

WOMEN

| HEIGHT (In Shoes)† Feet Inches | Weight in Pounds (In Indoor Clothing)* | | |
|---|---|---|---|
| | SMALL FRAME | MEDIUM FRAME | LARGE FRAME |
| 4  10 | 102–111 | 109–121 | 118–131 |
| 4  11 | 103–113 | 111–123 | 120–134 |
| 5  0 | 104–115 | 113–126 | 122–137 |
| 5  1 | 106–118 | 115–129 | 125–140 |
| 5  2 | 108–121 | 118–132 | 128–143 |
| 5  3 | 111–124 | 121–135 | 131–147 |
| 5  4 | 114–127 | 124–138 | 134–151 |
| 5  5 | 117–130 | 127–141 | 137–155 |
| 5  6 | 120–133 | 130–144 | 140–159 |
| 5  7 | 123–136 | 133–147 | 143–163 |
| 5  8 | 126–139 | 136–150 | 146–167 |
| 5  9 | 129–142 | 139–153 | 149–170 |
| 5  10 | 132–145 | 142–156 | 152–173 |
| 5  11 | 135–148 | 145–159 | 155–176 |
| 6  0 | 138–151 | 148–162 | 158–179 |

Source of basic data: Build Study, 1979, Society of Actuaries and Association of Life Insurance Medical Directors of America, 1980.
Copyright 1983 Metropolitan Life Insurance Company.

## WEIGHT REDUCTION DIET

Weight loss depends on (1) calories you do not eat and (2) calories you burn up during exercise. A low-calorie diet must be combined with exercise that increases calorie expenditure; otherwise you will not be able to prevent weight gain, which often occurs three to six months after stopping a low-calorie diet. It is best to lose slowly and plan your strategy over a one-year period. Therefore, try to lose two to four pounds per month, that is, twenty-four to forty-eight pounds over one year.

The body of an obese individual is programmed to form fat and store it. In addition, cells slow down and you burn fewer calories than normal. Your metabolic rate is slower than normal. When you go on a crash diet, your metabolic thermostat is turned down to get by on less food. Start your exercise program first, and after a month of walking one to two miles daily and climbing two to three flights of stairs four times daily, increase the exercise and then start your diet. Remember that a brisk two-mile walk in thirty minutes burns about 200 calories.

All weight reduction diets entail a major reduction in simple carbohydrate foods (sugar and starchy foods), which break down in the body to glucose (sugar). Therefore, you need to make a list of all such foods and reduce them by 50 to 75 percent (one half to three quarters) of your usual intake. I have not printed such a list, since they are readily available in most diet books.

All diets that are proven to cause sustained weight loss over a period of years depend on a reduced intake of calories. Therefore, calories do count. Don't let anyone tell you otherwise.

Your cells and muscles need energy to carry out their work. Energy is measured in calories. The body cells are like light bulbs. A bulb lights up when it receives enough electrical energy. The cells derive energy from chemical reactions involving glucose, oxygen, hydrogen, and high-energy phosphate bonds. The body needs glucose because it is one of the chief sources of energy—calories. The following example should help you understand weight loss and calories. Young diabetics lose a considerable amount of weight. Why? Insulin is required to transport glucose from the blood across the cell membrane to reach inside the cell to interact with other chemicals and so produce energy. When insulin is absent, glucose cannot get into the cells. Therefore, glucose reaches high levels in the blood and is passed out in the urine. The cells require energy to accomplish their particular function. When glucose is not present, the cells use fat as a source of energy. Thus, fat throughout the body is mobilized and broken down, resulting in marked weight loss, twenty to thirty pounds in two to three months.

Weight loss will be achieved if you reduce your calorie intake to 1,000 calories daily and burn up some calories by exercise. It is possible to eat attractive, appetizing meals and lose weight. Consider the following points in preparing your meals:

1. A meal containing high protein and low-to-moderate fat content as detailed in the "Sensible Heart Diet" is advisable. (see page 29)

2. Reduce intake of high-calorie foods: carbohydrate consisting of refined sugars and refined starches. Remember that alcohol, mixes, and beer contain calories.

3. Carbohydrate foods that have calories and can still be taken liberally include those containing high fiber. Foods with high fiber content allow you to eat a large meal; therefore, you feel satisfied. Most of the material stays longer in the stomach but is not digested and thus not absorbed into the blood. Your meal may have more calories, but you absorb only about half the amount of calories. I agree that high-fiber diets have a definite role in weight reduction plans. High-fiber foods include: wheat bran, green peas, chick peas, split peas, beans, corn, all vegetables, and fruits—in particular apples, pears, plums, nectarines, and the like, since the skin containing high fiber is eaten. Note that you can use whole grain flours to make your bread, pizzas, pastas, or muffins.

For further information on high-fiber foods and meal plans, the reader can consult Audrey Eyton's *The F-Plan Diet*.[54] However, I must issue a word of caution: Every intervention, be it type of diet or treatment, must be done in moderation. Importantly, I must draw your attention to the high Vitamin K content of certain high fiber foods often recommended— broccoli, turnip greens, spinach, and alfalfa. A high vitamin K intake may increase clotting factors in the blood. In addition, the occasional individual may have an increase in stools from once to three times daily, but this often normalizes. Very rarely anemia and bone loss (osteomalacia or osteoporosis) as well as a decreased absorption of minerals, such as calcium, zinc, or magnesium, may occur with a prolonged high-fiber reduction diet.[55] Therefore, do not over indulge.

*For those of you who have difficulty counting calories, simply try the following:*

1. *Reduce* your usual intake of the following foods by half (50%) to three quarters (75%). For example, four slices of bread daily becomes a maximum of two, or preferably one slice daily.
a. All white flour products: bread, pasta, spaghetti, macaroni, roti. Do not eat cakes, cookies, or pastries.
b. Rice.
c. Fried potatoes. However, one medium baked potato with skin can be eaten three times weekly.
d. Avoid fast foods and canned food because of their high calorie and salt content (see Table 2-2).
2. *Increase* your intake of:
a. All vegetables, including avocado, which is high in potassium and polyunsaturated fat despite its small content of saturated fat (Table 2-1).
b. All fruits.
c. Food with high fiber content; except broccoli, turnip greens, and alfalfa, which are rich in vitamin K. Small helpings of spinach or cabbage have less vitamin K and can be used.
d. Fish, chicken, veal, turkey.

In addition, if your blood cholesterol is greater than 250 mg, use only lean cuts of beef or steak twice weekly and only two eggs weekly. If your cholesterol is less than 220 mg, you can have a "nice" steak twice, shrimps once without a batter, and three to four eggs weekly.

The combination of foods allowed will afford pleasant-tasting meals that you can tolerate for months to years without depletion of protein, vitamins, or minerals. You will lose weight if you combine this diet with one hour of exercise at least five days weekly.

Obesity has been known to be a difficult problem to control. Motivation, willpower, and sacrifice are required. You may have greater success if you join a weight loss program or consult with a nutritionist regularly. Though a behavior modification program may help some,[57] to be really successful you need to find a weight loss program that will fit your particular lifestyle and weight loss goals.

You should not use diet plans that recommend low carbohydrates and advise a moderate-to-high fat intake. Some diet recipes reduce carbohydrates, but increase eggs, cheese, and meat products. Therefore, an increase in blood cholesterol may occur.

Studies have shown that liquid protein diets have certainly caused deaths and must not be used. Fifty deaths were reported in individuals who were using liquid protein diets. Seventeen of these individuals were known to be healthy, but developed abnormal heart rhythms while on the liquid protein diet.[58] However, no deaths occurred in a well-supervised study in which about 4,000 individuals were given an adequate amount (70 g) of first-class protein daily, along with a very low calorie diet.[58]

# DIABETES

There is no doubt that diabetes causes damage to arteries, especially those of the coronary, kidney, and leg vessels. Diabetes affects 2 to 3 percent of the North American population and is therefore not considered as major a risk factor as hypertension, which affects more than 20 percent of the population. This 2 percent does not include individuals found to have mild elevation of blood sugar and those informed that they have a touch of diabetes or glucose intolerance. This situation of mild glucose intolerance or possible mild chemical diabetes is not proven to carry the high risk of true diabetes. Many diabetics also have an increase in blood cholesterol and triglycerides. Atherosclerosis is commonly found and is due to the combination of high cholesterol, as well as damage to the arteries by the diabetic process.

In the past, the diabetic diet reduced carbohydrates and allowed a liberal intake of fats. An increase of fat in the diet increases blood cholesterol. Improved diet plans along with the techniques to achieve more efficient control of blood sugar may result in a reduction in cardiovascular complications. This hypothesis needs to be confirmed by further studies.

## TRIGLYCERIDES

Carbohydrate foods are converted in the body to glucose and triglycerides, and most overweight individuals have an increase in blood triglyceride level. Excess alcohol consumption and diabetes are well known to cause marked elevations in triglycerides. Fortunately, weight reduction and exercise rapidly decrease blood triglycerides. Normal values are 50 to 200 mg/dL, but values up to 300 mg should cause no panic. Elevations of 400 to 2,000 mg are commonly due to obesity or alcohol, and rarely, a genetic defect.

If your triglycerides are elevated, the first step is to repeat the estimation a few weeks later. No food or drink except water should be taken for fourteen hours prior to the test; otherwise a false elevation will be obtained. If they remain elevated higher than 300 mg, a weight-reduction diet low in carbohydrates and alcohol along with regular moderate exercise will cause a 20 to 33 percent decrease over a few months. Hypertriglyceridemia (high triglyceride blood level), unlike high blood cholesterol, responds extremely well to diet or drugs. In a few patients, if levels remain above 500 mg after six months of nondrug therapy, your doctor may prescribe a relatively safe drug, gemfibrozil, 600 mg twice daily. This drug markedly decreases triglycerides with mild lowering of cholesterol and causes a significant increase in HDL "good" cholesterol.

Hypertriglyceridemia is not considered a significant risk factor for the development of coronary heart disease. When a triglyceride level greater than 800 mg is combined with an elevation of LDL cholesterol and an HDL cholesterol level of less than 30 mg, the situation warrants treatment with diet and gemfibrozil.

# ALCOHOL

Alcohol is a central nervous system and heart muscle (myocardial) depressant. In acute experiments, eight ounces of alcohol given to healthy students over a two-hour period decreased the amount of blood the heart pumped into the arteries (cardiac output) by 33 percent. Patients with enlarged hearts or previous heart failure should not take alcohol, since it decreases the force of heart muscle contraction and can cause heart failure.

High consumption of alcohol of any type, beer or liquor, for several years can cause a severe weakening of and damage to the heart muscle, and this leads to severe enlargement of the heart and heart failure (heart muscle disease—cardiomyopathy). Fortunately, the condition is extremely rare. Low-to-moderate consumption of alcohol in healthy individuals or in patients with coronary heart disease without heart failure does not increase the risk of heart attack. Two to three ounces of alcohol consumed daily can increase HDL cholesterol levels by 5 to 10 percent, and whether this modest rise can be protective is not proven and remains controversial. Importantly, HDL consists of several fractions: $HDL_1$, $HDL_2$, and $HDL_3$. Recent studies indicate that alcohol does not increase $HDL_2$ "good" cholesterol levels but increases $HDL_3$ cholesterol, which does not appear to protect the arteries.

The message is this: If you are in the habit of consuming two ounces of alcohol daily, you may continue, but note that an increase to more than three ounces causes no further increase in HDL cholesterol. The evidence is premature, and if you do not drink, I agree with the experts who feel that it is foolhardy to commence. Remember that more than three ounces of alcohol daily can elevate blood pressure in susceptible individuals.

# VITAMINS

Vitamins E and $B_6$ are of no value in the treatment or prevention of heart disease, including heart attacks. The claims made by a few researchers many years ago have not been substantiated.

## ESTROGEN HORMONES

Normally menstruating women who are not on the birth control pill are protected from heart attacks. At age forty, the incidence of heart attack in men is twenty to one over women; at age fifty, about ten to one; at age sixty, about two to one; at age seventy-five, about one to one. Of 2,873 women who were followed for twenty-four years in the Framingham Study, no fatal or nonfatal heart attacks occurred in premenopausal women.[59] Heart attacks occurred in postmenopausal women. The exact reason for this protection remains unknown and debatable. It would seem that a decrease in endogenous estrogens formed in the body increases the risks. However, this is difficult to prove. It is difficult to explain why endogenous estrogens protect premenopausal women from coronary heart disease, but not from the development of atherosclerosis of the cerebral vessels, which can result in strokes. In addition, in clinical trials on men who had a heart attack and were given estrogens, recurrent or fatal heart attacks were not prevented.[60] However, the dose of estrogen used was very high (2.5 to 5 mg daily), and cardiovascular death rates were higher in patients receiving the higher dose. Since it is known that high doses of estrogen predispose an individual to blood clotting, the results of that study are not surprising. The protection that may occur with the use of a small dose of conjugated estrogen (.3 to 0.625 mg) has not been tested.

Menopausal and postmenopausal treatment with low-dose estrogens (0.3 to 0.6 mg) does not increase the risk of coronary heart disease and there is some evidence that cardiovascular risk may be decreased.[61] However, if a progestin, which contains the female hormone progesterone, or its derivatives is added to conjugated estrogen, the risk of stroke and heart attack can be slightly increased. If you need to take estrogen for menopausal symptoms, it is advisable to take 0.625 mg of conjugated estrogen for six to twelve months, then 0.3 mg for three to twelve months or longer if directed by your doctor. A progestin is not required if you have had a hysterectomy. If you have not had a hysterectomy, a progestin once daily for seven days is given by some gynecologists who believe that this might decrease the risk of uterine cancer due to estrogen therapy. However, this remains controversial. The problem of adding a progestin is a slightly increased risk of coronary heart disease; a possible inconvenience is withdrawal bleeding.

The oral contraceptive pill contains a mixture of estrogen and a progestin. The latter causes the menstrual bleeding on stopping the estrogen. The birth control pill increases the risk of heart attacks, mainly in women older than age thirty-five who are cigarette smokers.[62] The higher the estrogen and progestin content, the higher the alteration in LDL cholesterol and clotting factors. If you are over age thirty-five and smoke, do not take the birth control pill. If you are age forty or over, smoker or nonsmoker, do not take the birth control pill; let him have a vasectomy or seek alternative methods! At any age, if you take the pill and smoke, there is a slight increased risk of clots in the veins of the legs, the rare possibility of a stroke, and a very rare occurrence of heart attack. If you must use the birth control pill, use a very low dose of estrogen and do not smoke; your risk will then be minimal, whereas if you are age thirty-five and smoke, you have about a 1 in 1,000 chance of stroke or clots in the leg veins and about 1 in 10,000 chance of having a heart attack.

## TYPE A BEHAVIOR

Type A individuals have an impatient, time-conscious, achievement-striving personality, and often seek out a hectic environment that provokes undue stress. Leisure brings a feeling of guilt, since their lives are an everlasting struggle against time, toward achievement and recognition. The Type A takes on a project, including simple reading, with a certain violence. Speech is often harsh, explosive, or aggressive. When stressed, Type A individuals have been shown to release more adrenaline and noradrenaline and to have a greater rise in blood pressure than Type B's. Type B people are easygoing, able to relax, and rarely carry work home or set deadlines. Most of us are mixtures of Type A and B. It is difficult for a Type A person to change, but with expert assistance, modification of lifestyle is possible.

Friedman and Rosenman have defined and established the concept of the Type A behavior pattern.[63, 64] They emphasized that if you have Type A behavior, you have an increased risk of coronary heart disease. Several studies have confirmed that a relationship does exist between Type A behavior and risk of coronary heart disease. This occurs in both men and women independent of high blood cholesterol, hypertension, and smoking. The National Heart Lung Blood Institute has accepted the evidence regarding Type A behavior and increased risk of coronary heart disease.[65]

However, the question of Type A behavior and increased risk of coronary heart disease remains controversial. The large Multiple Risk Factor Intervention Study[21] and a small British study did not show any relationship. A study reported in the *New England Journal of Medicine* in March 1985 found no relationship between Type A behavior and mortality from coronary heart disease in patients who had had a heart attack and were followed for three years.[66] Commencing two weeks after their heart attack, 510 patients were followed. At the end of three years, death rate was not related to behavior, whether Type A or Type B. The mean Type A score did not differ significantly from the score of those who survived.[66]

Note that I did not discuss Type A behavior under the section on stress, since they represent two independent factors.

# CHAPTER 8

# PREVENTION OF BLOOD CLOTS (CORONARY THROMBOSIS)

## WHY AND WHEN DO BLOOD CLOTS OCCUR?

The cause of a fatal or a nonfatal heart attack in 90 percent of the cases is a blood clot in a coronary artery (coronary thrombosis).[2] The clot often occurs on the surface of a plaque of atheroma which partially obstructs the lumen of the coronary artery. Patients may have many large atheromatous plaques and yet not develop a clot over a five- to fifteen-year period. There is no test presently available and none forthcoming to tell us when and where a clot will occur. This is the $64,000 question. If we can fly to the moon, you would think that such a question can be answered.

Cholesterol, hypertension, and cigarette smoking have little to do with the clotting of blood; therefore, we must look elsewhere. I am convinced that unless we do something to help the population at risk to prevent a blood clot from forming in the coronary arteries, we will not have a major reduction in fatal and nonfatal heart attacks.

Recently cardiologists have started to use drugs to dissolve clots in the coronary artery. In many centers in North America, when a patient is admitted with a heart attack within three hours of onset of chest pain, a special test (coronary arteriography) is done, and this test locates the clot in a coronary artery.

87

The doctor will inject drugs that have recently been shown to be capable of dissolving a freshly formed clot. However, when a clot prevents blood from supplying part of the heart muscle, this area of the heart muscle cells dies within a half to one hour, and dissolving the clot may not really help because it is too late. Therefore, we should try to prevent the clot from forming.

The medical profession has spent billions of dollars on studies dealing with the risk factors, but very little has been done in the area of prevention of blood clots.

Small particles, platelets, are present in the blood and circulate as elliptical flat disks. Platelets are the first defense of the body against excessive bleeding. At the site of bleeding, platelets accumulate and stick together to form a clump to plug the ooze of blood. When the platelets clump together, other clotting factors come into play with the final conversion of a blood protein, fibrinogen, which turns into a mesh of fibrin strands that traps red cells and additional platelets, thus forming a firm clot.

Blood clots are believed to occur in the coronary artery because of the following:

1. Platelets become sticky when they come in contact with the damaged lining of blood vessels. Platelets interact with the damaged surfaces, and chemicals that are produced at the site cause the platelets to clump and form a clot. Chemicals in the body that cause platelets to clump or sludge include collagen from the damaged vessel wall, adrenaline, and a very powerful platelet-clumping chemical called thromboxane $A_2$.

2. Platelets are most sticky when they are newly released from the bone marrow. This may occur four to fourteen days after any type of surgery. For example, there is a higher incidence of clots in veins of the legs after surgical operations. The lack of movement of the legs causes a slowing of the circulation in veins and increases the chances of a clot in the deep veins of the legs.

3. Mild cooling and chilling of the body without hypothermia can lead to an increase in the total number and stickiness of platelets and may increase clotting.[67]

4.   During stress, adrenaline and other chemicals produced increase the number and stickiness of platelets, which may clump on to atheromatous plaques.

5.   Certain foods, especially a high-fat meal, increase the stickiness of platelets and influence other blood-clotting factors, but to a small extent.

6.   Atheromatous plaques produce turbulence and slow the blood flow in the coronary artery. The force of blood and increases in blood pressure can cause fissures or ulceration of plaques to occur. Platelets stick to these areas on the plaque and can start clot formation.

7.   Nicotine and carbon monoxide, which are by-products of cigarette smoking, increase platelet stickiness and may be important factors.

8.   Some foods have a high vitamin K content and increase the concentration of a clotting factor made in the liver (prothrombin). In addition, fibrinogen, the final protein involved in the formation of clots, is manufactured in the liver, and it has been shown that the mean fibrinogen concentration and viscosity in the blood is increased in patients who have had heart attacks.[68] Thus I believe that certain foods other than those involved in elevating blood cholesterol may be important in increasing or decreasing clot formation.

## NONDRUG TREATMENT

1.   I strongly recommend the following dietary measures:
a.   Eat less fatty meals, thereby reducing your saturated fat intake.
b.   Try to increase the intake of foods that may prevent blood clotting; in particular, onions, garlic, and foods containing linoleic and eicosapentaenoic acids, such as fish and cod liver oil. The latter polyunsaturated acid in the diet of fish-eating Japanese and Eskimos prevents clumping of platelets and has favorable effects on the blood clotting system.[12, 13] The aforementioned foods decrease platelet clumping as well as

increase vessel wall prostacyclin (prostaglandin), a compound that helps to keep the lining of the artery clean. Increase your consumption of fish, for example, mackerel and salmon, which have a high content of the aforementioned polyunsaturated fatty acids.

c. Avoid or use sparingly: alfalfa, turnip greens, and broccoli, which are very high in vitamin K, and lettuce, cabbage, and spinach, which have a moderate content. The concentration of prothrombin, a blood-clotting factor, can be increased by foods containing high vitamin K content.

2. Discontinue smoking cigarettes.
3. Learn to handle stress. An increase in the viscosity of the blood can increase the risk of clotting. Stress can increase the viscosity of blood as well as activate the platelet-clumping reaction described earlier.

## DRUG TREATMENT

1. Aspirin
2. Dipyridamole
3. Sulfinpyrazone
4. Ticlopidine
5. Anticoagulants

The four drugs listed first prevent platelet clumping (aggregation). They are not blood thinners (anticoagulants) and do not cause spontaneous bleeding.

### Aspirin

Aspirin blocks an enzyme (cyclo-oxygenase) within the blood platelets and prevents the formation of a substance, thromboxane $A_2$, which causes clumping of platelets. A dose of aspirin as low as 75 mg daily, a quarter of an ordinary aspirin, is capable of blocking the formation of thromboxane $A_2$. A dose of 325 mg (one ordinary aspirin) stops platelet clumping, and the effects last from one to two days. This reaction has been documented in man. However, several clinical trials in patients who have had heart attacks treated with aspirin did not show a reduction in deaths over a one- to two-year period. Unfortunately, such trials utilized large doses of aspirin, 650 to 1,800 mg daily, and we now know that large doses of aspirin block enzymes in the vessel walls called prostaglandins (prostacyclin), which normally help to keep the vessel wall clean and dilated. In order to obtain reliable answers, patients included in clinical trials, must be similar; i.e., one must study apples only and not apples mixed with oranges. Patients who are alive six months after a heart attack have a good outlook (prognosis) and those after twelve months have a greater chance of surviving five to ten years—an excellent prognosis. However, the large, well-run clinical trials utilizing aspirin studied patients who had suffered a heart attack from one to eighteen months prior to the commencement of aspirin treatment and this is not a good statistical approach. Thus, we can't exclude the possibility that a small dose such as a quarter to a maximum of one aspirin daily may prevent recurrence of heart attacks, especially if commenced a few days after the heart attack.

A study in patients with unstable angina showed that aspirin (325 mg daily) reduced the rate of fatal and nonfatal heart attacks by 50 percent.[69] I advise patients with coronary heart disease to take a 325 mg coated or baby aspirin daily.

## Dipyridamole

Supplied: Tablets: 50, 75 mg.
Dosage: 50 to 75 mg three times daily one hour before meals.

This drug is not useful when used alone, but in combination with aspirin, has been shown to reduce the incidence of clotting of coronary artery bypass grafts (CABG). In animal experiments, the drug has been shown to be effective in preventing platelet clumping. Rats stressed with electric shocks developed platelet clumping in the coronary arteries, which produced small areas of damage to the heart muscle (myocardial infarcts). This damage can be prevented in more than 80 percent of animals when pretreated with dipyridamole. Aspirin and sulfinpyrazone have similar effects.

During the 1970s a clinical trial called the Paris-1 Study evaluated the usefulness of dipyridamole combined with aspirin in about 2,000 patients who had had heart attacks. This study cost about $20 million to complete, but unfortunately included patients with old and very old heart attacks, that is, ranging from six months to three years. Only patients with less than a six-month-old heart attack showed a significant reduction in death rate, but this is not acceptable scientific evidence.

The combination of dipyridamole and aspirin was reevaluated in a 1980 to 1984 clinical trial. Three thousand patients were treated within thirty days of their heart attacks and followed for two years.

The combination was not of value in preventing deaths due to heart attacks, but caused a 37 percent reduction in the recurrence of heart attacks. The combination of aspirin and dipyridamole prevents formation of blood clots in vein grafts of patients who have had a coronary artery bypass graft. The drug has been proven to be useful when given for one year following coronary artery bypass surgery. Some surgeons may advise you to take the combination of aspirin and dipyridamole for several years. Dipyridamole is not useful when used without aspirin.

## Sulfinpyrazone

Sulfinpyrazone has been shown to reduce the incidence of fatal and nonfatal heart attacks including sudden death when given to patients from the seventh day after a heart attack for six months.[70] The U.S. Food and Drug Administration (FDA) did not approve this drug for general use because of minor discrepancies in the methods used in the trial.

## Ticlopidine

An investigational drug, ticlopidine, inhibits platelet clumping, and can decrease the frequency of chest pain as well as correct abnormal ECG changes in patients with attacks of angina due to coronary heart disease. These studies serve to implicate platelets as a major culprit in the causation of complications of coronary heart disease including fatal or nonfatal heart attacks or angina.

## Anticoagulants (warfarin)

Anticoagulants (blood thinners) are not effective in preventing a first or recurrent heart attack. They were used for this purpose from 1955 and abandoned from about 1968. They are used successfully for the treatment of clots in:

1. Leg veins
2. The lungs (pulmonary embolism)
3. The heart chambers (atrium or ventricle), especially if such clots move from the heart and block an artery elsewhere in the body such as in the legs or brain. Fortunately, the latter occurrence is rare.

## CONCLUSION

Aspirin is useful but needs further clinical trials to document beneficial effects as well as the minimum effective daily dosage. Until we have this information, the majority of doctors will not advise patients who have had a heart attack to take one aspirin daily. Unfortunately, we may never have further clinical trials, since the previous aspirin trials cost more than $40 million. In addition, low-dose aspirin was not studied. The patients studied had had heart attacks from one to twenty-four months before they began taking aspirin; therefore, any beneficial effects were likely missed.

A clinical trial done in Canada and reported in the New England Journal of Medicine, November 1985, confirms the beneficial effects of aspirin in patients with unstable angina. If your doctor says that you have unstable angina, a very severe form of angina, you should discuss with your doctor the possibility of taking one aspirin, preferably enteric-coated, once daily since this may prevent you from having a heart attack.

# CHAPTER 9

---

# BETA-BLOCKING DRUGS (BETA-BLOCKERS) TO PREVENT HEART ATTACKS AND DEATH

The surfaces of cells in various organs and tissues have receptor sites. Hormones and other chemicals react at their respective receptor site to bring about a particular action in the cell. Adrenaline and noradrenaline are called catecholamines and are released from sympathetic nerve endings and as hormones from the adrenal glands. They have their major actions on receptor sites called beta-receptors. Stimulation of the sympathetic-adrenal system during danger or severe stress, for example, causes an outpouring of adrenaline and noradrenaline into the blood circulation and at nerve endings. Catecholamines are stimulants and cause an increase in the force of contraction of the heart, and increase heart rate, blood pressure, and blood sugar. An outpouring of catecholamines is necessary to prepare the body for a fight-or-flight response. Therefore, we need this surge of adrenaline if we have to flee from a charging bull. While adrenaline and noradrenaline have good effects, in excess they have bad effects and cause overcharging of the cardiovascular system.

It is well documented that during a heart attack large quantities of noradrenaline are released into the heart muscle and can precipitate abnormal heart rhythms, in particular, ventricular fibrillation, during which the heart "quivers," i.e., stops beating, and death occurs. Adrenaline causes an increase in heart rate and an increase in blood pressure and thus causes the heart to work harder. Because a coronary artery is blocked during a heart attack, the increased work with less oxygen available causes further damage to the heart muscle and increases the size of the muscle damage, thus causing a larger heart attack.

By definition, beta-blockers block beta-receptors. Structurally they resemble the catecholamines (adrenaline and noradrenaline) and block the action of these catecholamines at their receptor sites. As a result, heart rate is reduced, resulting in a slower pulse; the force of heart muscle contraction is reduced; a lowered blood pressure, a stabilized heart rhythm, and a significant reduction in the occurrence of ventricular fibrillation occurs. Beta-blockers cause the heart muscle to work less, thus requiring a reduced amount of oxygen, and in time of oxygen lack, such as during a heart attack, this action can be life-saving. Because of the reduction in the oxygen requirement of the heart muscle, the beta-blocking drugs are effective in preventing the chest pain of angina pectoris. Since patients with angina have a high risk of developing a heart attack over ensuing years, beta-blockers are important for both pain and prevention. In addition, beta-blockers alter clotting factors and thus may prevent a buildup of sludge, or clotting of blood, without causing bleeding.

An increase in adrenaline such as produced during stress or vigorous exercise causes an increase in (1) the number and stickiness of blood platelets, (2) a clotting factor (factor VIII, hemophilic factor), and (3) viscosity of the blood. Beta-blockers block the effect of adrenaline and noradrenaline, and thus may inhibit a blood clot.

Well-run clinical trials have documented that beta-blockers significantly prevent death in patients who are given the drug from the first week of the heart attack and for an additional two years.[1, 71]

In the superbly well run Norwegian study, 1,884 patients were divided into two groups. Randomly, 942 patients were started on a beta-blocker, timolol, seven days after their heart attack. The other group of 942 patients received a placebo. At the end of two years follow-up, the treated group had a 35 percent reduction in heart death, 28 percent reduction in new heart attack, and 65 percent reduction in sudden death.[1] The results are statistically significant. The American Beta Blocker Heart Attack trial gave similar if not just as impressive results.[71]

It is interesting to note the good effect of beta-blockers on the arterial system. The thousands of miles of arteries are constantly under pressure from the pulsatile force and velocity of blood as well as blood pressure. Atherosclerosis is commonly seen where arteries divide, especially when they do so near right angles. Beta-blockers reduce blood pressure as well as the force and velocity of blood flow at these points of mechanical stress and provide some protection from vessel wall injury. This favorable effect is of paramount importance in patients with high blood pressure. Mechanical injury from the velocity and force of blood is the prime cause of vessel wall injury, which leads to atherosclerosis, dissection of the plaques of atheroma, and subsequent thrombosis, as well as rupture of a vessel.

The name of the game is *preventing heart attacks, as well as preventing death*. Beta-blockers and aspirin are the only drugs that are proven by studies in man to prevent death from heart attack.[1, 71, 72] In addition, about 425,000 heart attack patients survive to leave hospitals in the United States annually, and about 80,000 of these patients will have another heart attack in the ensuing year. Beta-blockers can prevent a heart attack in approximately 25 percent (20,000) of these patients. It is worth your while to get this protection, provided there is no contraindication to the use of a beta-blocking drug.

The clinical trials that substantiate the good effects of beta-blockers in the post–heart attack patients and the reason why some doctors are reluctant to prescribe them are given in Chapter 10, "How to Deal with Heart Attacks."

The beta-blockers that are available and used to prevent fatal or nonfatal heart attacks and in the management of angina or hypertension are given in Chapters 10 and 11.

# CONCLUSIONS

Prevention of fatal or nonfatal heart attacks requires a lot of work on the part of doctors and the public. It is your body, and you can work to protect it from the big killers: heart attack, hypertension, and stroke. Our discussion should indicate to you that there are no easy answers. Reviews given in magazines and in some books for the public are often superficial or full of gimmicks and quick fixes that mislead the public.

*Prevention* requires:

1.  Efficient *control* of the *risk factors*—hypertension, high blood cholesterol, smoking, and stress.
2.  More attention must be given to the *prevention of blood clotting* so as to prevent coronary thrombosis. This goal requires:

    a.  The favorable adjustment to certain foods that can prevent the formation of clots.
    b.  The use of drugs that decrease blood clotting without causing bleeding, for example, half to one aspirin daily. Similar and more effective drugs are being tested and will soon become available; so there is hope.

3.  *Beta-blocking drugs* are advisable for those at moderate to high risk, i.e., patients with heart attacks, angina, or hypertension.

I strongly recommend that you use this information in conjunction with the advice of your doctor to gain maximum protection and thus prevent your heart attacks.

# PART II

# MANAGEMENT OF CORONARY HEART DISEASE

**CHAPTER 10**

---

# HOW TO DEAL WITH HEART ATTACKS

It is of utmost importance that you learn to recognize the signs and symptoms of a heart attack. Thus you may help yourself, your spouse, or a friend to receive quick and successful treatment. Consider that someday you may save a life, especially your own.

In the majority of individuals, the cause of a heart attack is a clot (thrombosis) in one of the coronary arteries. The clot can be dissolved by special drugs that I will discuss later in this chapter. However, for this treatment to be effective, it must be given within three hours and a maximum of four hours from the onset of the symptoms of a heart attack, that is, three hours from the onset of chest pain, which is the most common symptom. Beyond four hours, the chance of success with this treatment is remote, since the heart muscle cells become irreversibly damaged and die between two and five hours after the blood supply has been cut off. Therefore, I strongly advise you to learn the symptoms and signs of a heart attack. If these suggest a heart attack, you should go rapidly to the emergency room of a hospital that has facilities to dissolve clots in the coronary artery.

## SYMPTOMS AND SIGNS OF A HEART ATTACK

Symptoms are often typical and easy to recognize. However, in some patients, symptoms can be so varied that both the patient and the doctor can be misled. People have unique feelings and sensations and use different words to describe similar symptoms. Heart attacks vary a great deal in their severity, and patients are not all alike. Thus, the characteristics of pain and accompanying symptoms can be very different from one individual to another. I will discuss the feelings that an individual may perceive or experience and give clues as to the diagnosis using the following categories:

1.  The type or character of pain: what does it feel like?
2.  The location of the pain.
3.  The severity and duration of the pain.
4.  Warning attacks.
5.  Associated symptoms.
6.  What other conditions cause chest pain and can mimic a heart attack?
7.  Are age, sex, family history, and risk factors important in making a diagnosis of heart attack?

## The Type or Character of Pain: What Does It Feel Like?

The patient may have difficulty describing the type of pain or peculiar discomfort or distress. Some words used by various patients to describe the discomfort may seem similar, but I will list them so that you can learn to recognize the peculiar sensation:

1.  *Crushing*—compressing pain or a heaviness over the chest. The pain is most often described as "a crushing pain across my chest." Or the patient states that it feels like a very heavy weight or bar is resting on the center of the chest, especially over the breastbone (sternum) or, "It feels as if someone is crushing or walking on my chest."
2.  *Viselike*—tightness, squeezing, constricting. It feels as if the chest is in a vise or as if a tight metal band is being pulled around the chest. The constricting feeling is often described as a tightness. The patient tries to describe the tightness by clenching a fist. Many patients, before being asked to describe the pain, are

observed to be clenching one or both fists, one of which may lie over the breastbone in the center of the chest or upper part of the stomach. In the majority of cases, the pain is felt as if it were coming from the undersurface of the breastbone but an exact description will follow outlining the severity of the pain and where in the chest the pain is felt.

3.   *Strangling*—a disagreeable choking, strangling, sickening feeling in the center and across the chest. This type of sensation can occur in patients with anxiety states and may not be due to a heart attack. However, this strangling quality is very important because it resembles the discomfort in patients with angina pectoris. Patients with angina can develop chest discomfort mainly on exertion and this pain is due to a lack of blood supply to the heart muscle. If the strangling sensation comes on at rest and lasts for more than thirty minutes and especially if it is accompanied by the associated symptoms of a heart attack, you should seek attention.

4.   *Burning-like indigestion*. A burning discomfort or pain in the center of the chest, especially when accompanied by sweating or sensations listed under associated symptoms, must be taken seriously as it can be caused by a heart attack. Pain originating from the stomach is often burning in quality, but the associated symptoms serve to differentiate heart from stomach pain. For example, heart pain is very often associated with profuse sweating, whereas stomach pain rarely ever causes sweating.

5.   *Tearing, gripping pain*, as if the chest were being pulled apart from the breastbone.

6.   *Fullness in the chest*, as if it wanted to explode, may be a symptom of a heart attack but it can be due to pain originating from the stomach or gullet (esophagus), for example, gas pains, or to reflux esophagitis.

7.   *Just a discomfort*. The patient may not perceive the sensation as pain but as a mild to moderate discomfort. Such a discomfort is a common feature and must not be ignored, especially if associated signs and symptoms are present.

8. *Tingling, numbness, or heaviness* over the left or right arm may occur at the same time as the pain in the chest but rarely can be the only manifestation of a heart attack. However, there are many causes of such symptoms in the arms, especially pain from the nerves supplying the arms, muscular pain, or a small stroke, in which case, the hand and the arm will be very weak. A heart attack does not cause the arm or hand to become severely weak and it never causes a paralysis.

9. *A pointed, sharp, stabbing, sticking, knifelike pain* is seldom a manifestation of a heart attack. Such chest pain is often produced by other sources, such as the chest wall or the lungs, as in pleurisy and gas pains.

10. *Dizziness and/or severe weakness* commonly occurs along with the chest pain of a heart attack, but is rarely the only symptom.

11. *Nausea without vomiting or diarrhea,* if associated with pain in the chest or discomfort or shortness of breath, weakness, or dizziness, can be a symptom of a heart attack and rarely occurs without chest pain. In such a situation, associated shortness of breath points to a disturbance of the heart, rather than the stomach.

12. *Aching pain under the breastbone* or arm is occasionally described by patients.

I am sure you can recognize a dog from its bark and will not confuse this with a cat even if you are blindfolded. You will recognize a heart attack from the character of the chest pain and the company it keeps; that is, we need to associate the pain and the severity with the location and other associated symptoms commonly found with a heart attack.

## The Location of the Pain

In the majority of individuals, the pain of a heart attack is located in the center of the chest under the breastbone (retrosternal). The pain is more often located under the lower two-thirds of the breastbone (Figure 10-1).

Note that the heart projects out to the left side of the

## Figure 10-1  Common Sites of Heart Pain

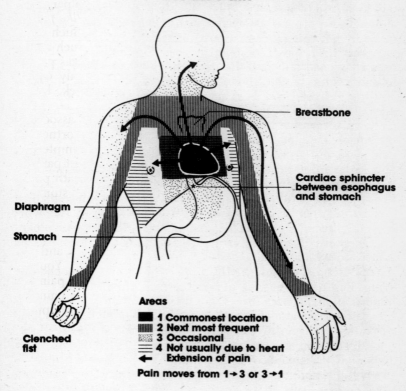

Breastbone

Cardiac sphincter between esophagus and stomach

Diaphragm

Stomach

Clenched fist

**Areas**

■ 1 Commonest location
▥ 2 Next most frequent
▦ 3 Occasional
≡ 4 Not usually due to heart
← Extension of pain

Pain moves from 1→3 or 3→1

breastbone and pain under/or outside of the nipple line rarely comes from a heart attack. I would like to draw your attention to the importance of the fist in the diagnosis of a heart attack. Many patients automatically use a clenched fist to indicate that the pain in the chest is a squeezing, tightness, or pressurelike sensation. When the pain is originating from the heart, the size of the area of pain or discomfort is usually the size of a fist and not less than two finger tips. If the area of pain or discomfort is one finger tip or less, it is very unlikely to arise from the heart, and if there are no associated symptoms, the pain is nearly certainly not coming from a heart attack.

The next most common area is the upper half of the breastbone and the pit of the stomach. Heart pain occurs mainly in the center of the chest, and doctors often use the term "central retrosternal chest pain" as being typical of a heart attack. Finally, pain from all three areas can move (radiate) up or down to involve the entire chest, the neck, the throat, and the lower jaw (not higher than the upper jaw) and commonly extend to the arms, the forearms, and the hands. Both arms may feel painful, heavy, numb, or tingly. Left arm discomfort is more common than right, and as shown in Figure 10-1, area 2, the inner aspect (ulnar side of the arm) is the commonest site of arm pain. Most of the arm or a small part such as the wrist may be the site of pain or discomfort without involvement of the chest. However, arm, jaw, or throat pain is usually associated with a simultaneous occurrence of pain in the chest. If pain is present only in the upper limb, the accompanying symptoms and signs of a heart attack then become very important in making the diagnosis. For example, if there is associated shortness of breath, nausea, and sudden generalized weakness, the arm pain can be the manifestation of a heart attack.

Heart pain can occur anywhere in the chest or upper abdomen, neck, jaw, or upper limbs. Pain below the level of the belly button (umbilicus) is not from the heart. In addition, the pain of a heart attack very rarely goes through to the back. If it does, it is usually the zone between the left shoulder blade and the spine. Pain present only in the area on both sides of a vertical line drawn through the nipple is most unlikely to be due to a heart attack (Figure 10-1). However, centrally located breastbone pain can radiate across the entire chest, that is, to the left and occasionally to the right of the nipple line and upward to the neck and jaw. Thus, while in some cases, the size of the area may be that of one to three clenched fists or the entire span of the palm and outstretched fingers, pain can spread to involve the entire front of the chest.

## The Severity and Duration of the Pain

The pain of a heart attack is variable in intensity. In about 50 percent of patients, it is described as severe pain. However, in about 10 percent of patients, it is very severe and unbearable. In about 20 percent of patients, the pain is a moderate pain that is not in itself distressing and may well be a mild discomfort not reaching the level of pain. In such patients, the associated symptoms are important, especially the feeling of anguish or fear of impending doom, which is common in patients who are having a heart attack. In about 10 percent of the cases, there is profound weakness, sweating, dizziness, nausea, or palpitations. In the remaining 10 percent of the cases, no symptoms occur and a heart attack is discovered only on subsequent routine electrocardiographic or autopsy examinations.

The duration of pain during a heart attack is usually more than thirty minutes and frequently one to four hours. A pain that lasts less than one minute and returns each time only to last a couple of minutes is usually not due to a heart attack, especially if there are no other associated symptoms. Pain lasting less than ten seconds, even when recurrent, is not due to a heart attack. The pain of angina usually lasts from one to five minutes and its maximum is fifteen minutes. If the pain is similar to the accustomed anginal pain but now lasts more than thirty minutes, especially if at rest, you must seriously consider the possibility of a heart attack.

Diabetics and patients over age seventy-five may have little or no pain during a heart attack. Thus, the elderly may get weakness or shortness of breath without chest pain. The pain of a heart attack can come on gradually over a half to one hour with increasing intensity that may remain steady for a few hours. It is usually a steady pain, not an on-and-off pain such as occurs with crampy stomach problems or gut pain that is usually described as colic (colicky or spasmodic pain). Importantly, after one to four hours, the pain of a heart attack may suddenly disappear never to return and the individual may feel fairly well. The patient may no longer be disturbed and can make the mistake of not going to an emergency room. Pain ceases as the heart muscle cells die when they are deprived of blood. *Dead muscle cells produce no pain.* The pain may disappear before reaching the emergency room. Or pain may be quickly relieved by morphine and not recur. Thus, the patient who does not understand the situation may wish to leave the emergency room or hospital. On rare occasions, pain may persist for six to twelve hours in three or four bouts each lasting a few hours, and between times, a dull pressure, tightness, heaviness, or ache remains somewhere in the center of the chest or areas described under location of heart pain.

## Warning Attacks

In about 20 to 30 percent of patients with a heart attack there is a "warning." It is present some time during the prior two weeks in patients who have chest pain (angina) and suddenly notice a change in the duration and frequency of the pain. Instead of pain lasting one to five minutes, the pain may last five to twenty minutes and is brought on with less activity and may finally occur at rest. This usually indicates that the angina is progressing or unstable. If the pain lasts longer than thirty minutes and is not relieved by two nitroglycerin tablets, it is likely due to a heart attack. However, if the pain lasts from fifteen to thirty minutes, it is likely due to unstable angina that can lead to a heart attack over the next few months. In such a situation, you can prevent a heart attack if you get proper attention.

In patients who are not known to have angina, pain may suddenly come on for the first time during a bout of unaccustomed exertion such as shoveling snow, pushing a car, hauling a boat, or running. Chest pain or discomfort may only last two to ten minutes and may be ignored only to return in full force within a few days. If pain occurs for only a few minutes, take special note if the pain is relieved within one to two minutes after stopping the precipitating activity. About 25 percent of such patients are likely to have a heart attack within the next month and these may be prevented by the combination of a beta-blocking drug and one aspirin daily. In addition, the electrocardiogram is usually normal in such patients when pain is absent. Thus, they are often sent away from the emergency room. However, this must not deter you from seeking appropriate expert medical care.

## Associated Symptoms

As discussed above, pain or discomfort of a heart attack is nearly always accompanied by one or more symptoms, which may help you or the doctor clarify the diagnosis. Therefore, identifying these associated symptoms is of vital importance.

1.  Sweating is often profuse for at least a few minutes. In particular, the forehead is usually covered with a cold sweat. Importantly, indigestion or stomach pains that can be confused with a heart attack do not usually cause profuse sweating. It is well known that sweating occurs during a fever as the temperature rises above 100°F (38°C). However, a heart attack does not cause a rise in body temperature until about the second day. Therefore, if you have sudden pain and definite fever, it is most unlikely to be due to a heart attack.

2.  Difficulty breathing is very common and may last for a few minutes. Persistence of shortness of breath for more than ten minutes suggests that blood and fluid are accumulating in the lungs due to heart failure and requires prompt attention. Shortness of breath must be distinguished from sighing respirations, which involve taking one or two deep breaths and completely exhaling. Sighing is a common occurrence in individuals who are under stress and can be due to tiredness, exhaustion, or anxiety. Difficulty in breathing can mean several things: You cannot take a deep breath because your chest hurts—for example, if a rib is fractured or an infection is present on the outer surface of the lung membrane (pleurisy). On movement of the chest wall,

lung pain is produced; therefore, a deep breath cannot be taken because it causes pain and the individual is forced to take shallow breaths. Shortness of breath is a different sensation and it means that you feel out of breath and you are forced to gasp and run after your breath, breathing rapidly and shallowly. The feeling is similar to that of running up four or five flights of stairs. Afterward, you are out of breath and have to breathe harder and quicker. During heart failure the lungs have extra water and blood and become very stiff, making a very deep breath impossible; therefore, the breathing tends to be a little shallow. When shortness of breath is due to heart trouble, it is made worse by lying flat and can improve a little if the individual sits up and dangles the legs. Some nervous and anxious individuals hyperventilate and this must be differentiated from true shortness of breath.

To reemphasize, the pain of a heart attack is not increased by taking a very deep breath, coughing, or sneezing.

3.   Virtually all patients with heart attacks have a feeling of impending doom. This fear and anxiety can provoke secretion of adrenaline and noradrenaline, which increases heart damage and may disturb the heart rhythm. The increase in adrenaline causes irritability of the dying heart muscle and triggers the production of extra beats and occasionally may result in ventricular fibrillation, during which the heart muscle does not contract but quivers. It is imperative that pain, fear, and anxiety be quickly relieved with adequate pain-relieving drugs such as morphine and with reassurance by a doctor. You will reassure yourself if you quickly reach a hospital where adequate facilities exist to relieve pain and combat your heart attack.

One of my patients, a male age forty-eight, had several typical symptoms during his heart attack: he suddenly experienced a disagreeable sensation in the chest, which increased to a heavy crushing sensation over and beneath the lower part of the breastbone. During the next ten to fifteen minutes, the pain felt like a heavy bar across the chest and within a few minutes spread to his left arm, which felt as heavy as lead. He was not known to have angina and therefore had no nitroglycerin available. However, he was over-come by a strange fear with a feeling that life was going to be extinguished. At this point, his pain had lasted about forty minutes, and was moderately severe but could not be described as unbearable. He was sweating profusely and upon further questioning, he admitted that it was his fear that prompted him to call the ambulance. It is true that many people are afraid of a heart attack and may develop anxiety. Many individuals with pain in different parts of the body may become a little anxious, but few feel as if they are strangling and this sensation seems to produce great fear and anxiety. Perhaps the body is trying to tell you to do something quickly about this feeling.

4.  Severe and sudden weakness may be associated with the chest discomfort in about one-third of patients with a heart attack. The heart muscle is damaged and cannot pump with maximum force. Less blood is ejected from the heart at each beat; therefore blood pressure falls and less blood reaches the brain. Thus, the patient may feel weak and feel like fainting. Transient loss of consciousness for a couple of minutes can occur but is uncommon. The blood pressure soon becomes restored to near normal because of the body's compensatory responses, and weakness improves. In a few patients with a large heart attack, the blood pressure remains very low and the weakness is profound (cardiogenic shock).

5.  Dizziness or lightheadedness may occur in some patients owing to a drop in blood pressure. Ringing in the ears (tinnitus) or severe rotational dizziness (vertigo) are not usually features of a heart attack.

6.  Nausea and occasionally vomiting accompanies the pain in a significant number of patients. Severe pain from any cause may precipitate vomiting, and pain relievers such as morphine usually increase nausea and vomiting. However, unaccustomed sudden nausea may occur instead of pain or chest discomfort. Thus, distressing nausea with sweating and shortness of breath should be considered due to a heart disturbance until proven otherwise.

7.  Restlessness. The pain or discomfort of a heart attack
    is not relieved by any particular position. The pain is
    not made better or worse by sitting, standing, lying, or
    rolling from side to side. The patient tries to achieve a
    comfortable position but finds none. Therefore, rest-
    lessness is common. Because pain is often vicelike
    (squeezing) and over the lower half of the breastbone,
    the individual is often seen with a clenched fist held
    against the breastbone. If the heart muscle is very
    weak and heart failure occurs during the heart attack,
    the individual is found to be short of breath and may
    be gasping. In such cases, some relief is obtained
    when the patient is propped up in bed. A cough may
    suddenly develop with the production of frothy pink or
    blood-stained sputum. If the condition is extremely
    bad, severe weakness with confusion and loss of con-
    sciousness may occur owing to a big fall in blood
    pressure, which results in severe lack of blood supply
    to the brain. When the heart muscle is suddenly weak-
    ened by a heart attack, the blood pressure may fall
    from 10 to 40 mm of Hg and the pulse may become
    rapid, thus in about half of the patients with heart
    attacks, the systolic blood pressure may fall from an
    average of 125 mm to less than 105 mm. However,
    during the next few hours, if the heart attack is not a
    very large one, the body's compensatory responses
    may be sufficient to increase the blood pressure to the
    normal systolic range for the individual. The fall in
    blood pressure caused by a heart attack often reduces
    the blood pressure of a hypertensive patient to normal
    so that medications for high blood pressure may not be
    required for several months and in some forever. I feel
    it is wise for all patients with known coronary heart
    disease and perhaps for all males over age forty and
    females over age fifty to invest in a blood pressure
    instrument. A doctor can teach you how to measure
    blood pressure and then you, your spouse, or a friend
    can take it every three months so that you know your
    average blood pressure reading (See "Measurement
    of Blood Pressure" in Chapter 13.) Thus, if you are
    worried about chest discomfort or indigestion that is

not relieved by an antacid and your systolic blood pressure falls more than 30 mm, this should prompt a visit to an emergency room. If you are in doubt because the discomfort seems to be in the stomach, an associated fall in blood pressure may warn you and save your life. On the other hand, since not all patients have a fall in blood pressure and the rare patient may have a mild increase in blood pressure because of pain and nervous reflexes, do not wait for a fall in blood pressure if chest pain with other associated symptoms is present; go to the emergency room.

I feel it is important for everyone over age thirty-five to learn how to determine the heart rate by feeling the pulse at the wrist. If during chest discomfort, the pulse decreases by twenty or increases by twenty when you are at rest, this is likely to be a warning of a heart attack. For example, if your resting pulse rate is usually in the range of seventy to eighty beats per minute and you suddenly find it at fifty to sixty beats per minute while having chest discomfort, the disturbance likely originates from the heart, especially if you are not on medication such as beta-blockers, which slow the pulse rate. A reduction in heart rate of ten or less is too small to be diagnostic.

If the back of the heart muscle is affected during the attack (inferior heart attack), the pulse usually slows. If the front part of the heart muscle is affected (anterior heart attack), the pulse usually increases by 20 to 40 beats per minute and can reach 100 to 120 beats per minute at rest.

I would strongly suggest that if you have coronary heart disease or if you are over forty, your home should be equipped with a blood pressure instrument and nitroglycerin should be available. Both are as essential as having a smoke detector or a fire extinguisher in the home. It is far more important to learn the symptoms and signs of a heart attack and the procedure for measuring your blood pressure and taking your pulse than it is to learn about cardiopulmonary resuscitation (CPR).

# WHAT OTHER CONDITIONS CAUSE CHEST PAIN AND CAN MIMIC A HEART ATTACK?

1. Indigestion and reflux esophagitis, haitus hernia, and esophageal spasm.
2. Lung infections: pleurisy and pneumonia.
3. Pericarditis.
4. Chest wall pain: originating from the muscles, ribs, intercostal nerves, or costo-chondral joints, or due to a common condition, costo-chondritis.
5. Arm pain, tingling, and numbness in the left or right upper limb.

Other causes are very rare and are not included so as not to confuse the reader. I do not intend to turn you into a doctor, but to give you clear pointers that can be of value.

You must be reassured that about half of the patients admitted to the hospital because of chest pain with the diagnosis of possible heart attack turn out not to have a heart attack. These patients usually have an unstable form of angina pectoris, chest wall pain, stomach problems (in particular, reflux esophagitis with esophageal spasm), and very rarely pericarditis. Occasionally no cause can be found.

## Indigestion and Stomach Problems

These problems, including esophageal pain due to reflux, are described in detail since they commonly occur and can mimic a heart attack. Those of you who have indigestion must know how to recognize this since you feel it 10 to 365 times per year and can quickly distinguish it from the symptoms or discomfort that may occur if a heart attack occurs. Pain of a heart attack can be present in the pit of the stomach (upper epigastrium) and the lower sternal area and may even be burning in type. Burning pain is more common with stomach and esophageal pain and relieved by antacids, but the burning caused by a heart attack is not relieved by antacids. Associated profuse sweating or shortness of breath points to a heart attack rather than stomach or esophageal pain. Pain from ulcers in the stomach does not cause sweating and is related to meals and is often relieved by antacids.

## Reflux Esophagitis and Hiatus Hernia

A sphincter is present at the junction of the esophagus and stomach (Figure 10-1). This cardiac sphincter closes tightly when an individual is at rest, but relaxes and opens in response to swallowing to allow food to enter the stomach. When you are not swallowing, the lower esophageal sphincter is tightly closed and prevents stomach contents such as hydrochloric acid and constituents of the bile from flowing backward into the lower esophagus (gastroesophageal reflux). In some individuals, either in response to a hernia of the stomach that protrudes into the chest along the lower esophagus (hiatus hernia), heredity, or aging, the sphincter becomes incompetent and opens during rest. It opens further if intra-abdominal pressure is increased during straining, stooping, or lifting heavy objects, or during pregnancy. Reflux is always worse within one hour of eating especially if excess fluids were taken. Importantly, a high-fat meal delays emptying of the stomach and reflux may last for hours rather than minutes. The reflux of acid and stomach contents such as pepsin, bile salts, and pancreatic enzymes causes a severe irritation and at times inflammation of the lower esophagus. The condition is called an esophagitis, which is similar to having an ulcer in the stomach. Distressing symptoms persist for many years and may result in narrowing (stricture) of the lower esophagus with difficulty in swallowing.

Reflux esophagitis commonly causes discomfort in the lower chest (retrosternal) as does heart attack or angina. The burning, pressurelike pain or discomfort can radiate along the entire breastbone to the back and sometimes the arm. Heartburn is common and regurgitation of bitter sour fluid or food, without vomiting, commonly occurs. Free acid reflux in the recumbent position can cause the patient to be awakened by the discomfort. Spicy and acid foods, especially citrus juice, coffee, and fatty meals increase the discomfort, which at times may be difficult to differentiate from a heart condition such as angina.

As mentioned earlier, a heart attack commonly causes profuse sweating and shortness of breath, whereas reflux esophagitis does not.

The diagnosis is easily made by X-ray. Using a barium swallow or a meal, the radiologist documents reflux of barium from the stomach into the esophagus. Tests are available to detect incompetence of the cardiac sphincter, and gastroscopy shows inflammation of the lower end of the esophagus with or without the presence of a hiatus hernia. A hernia often increases reflux, but the effect is variable. Reflux commonly occurs without the presence of hernia and may not occur when a hernia is present.

### Esophageal Reflux Is Relieved By:

a. Antacids.
b. Elevation of the head of the bed and refraining from lying down for at least two hours after a meal or a drink of liquid.
c. Avoidance of spicy foods, fatty foods, and acid liquids such as citrus juices.
d. Avoidance of bending and stooping and lifting, especially within one hour after meals.
e. Weight reduction.
f. Use of drugs such as metoclopramide, which increases the tone or competence of the cardiac sphincter.

## Esophageal Spasm

This condition is not as common as gastroesophageal reflux, but can closely mimic a heart attack and frequently occurs in patients who have esophageal reflux. It can occur at any age but is more common after age forty. The most common site of pain is behind the lower half of the breastbone and can radiate upward along the breastbone to the throat, jaw, back, or arms. Pain can be squeezing, dull, or sharp; moderate to severe; and last minutes to hours. Importantly, the pain can occur at night, the individual being awakened by moderately severe pain that can be mistaken for a heart attack. Pain may come on during or after a meal especially after a drink of cold liquid. Severe anxiety and stress can produce an attack. However, there may be no precipitating factors. In many patients with esophageal spasm, there is some difficulty in swallowing, and this can occur with or without the presence of pain. The diagnosis is usually confirmed by X-ray fluoroscopy during which the individual swallows liquid barium. Other confirmatory tests can be done by a gastroenterologist. Nitroglycerin may relieve the pain of esophageal spasm. As well, a calcium antagonist, nifedipine, which relieves muscle spasm, can sometimes abolish the pain of esophageal spasm. Antacids or warm milk may relieve the pain of esophageal spasm, but not that which arises from the heart.

## Lung Infections

Pneumonia may produce pain, and this is usually a sharp pain that is made worse by taking a very deep breath or coughing. The pain occurs because the outer membrane of the lung, the pleura, is involved in the inflammation, that is, a pleurisy. Usually there are fever, chills, and cough.

## Pericarditis

This is an inflammation of the outer membrane of the heart, which can be caused by a virus, a bacteria, or a heart attack. The pain is usually sharp, located over the lower breastbone or a little to the left of the breastbone, and is sometimes made worse by deep breathing when the pericardium and pleura are both involved. The pain is usually made worse by lying down and is quickly improved by sitting up and leaning forward. Three or four days after a heart attack, a few patients develop pericarditis. This resolves in a few days.

## Chest Wall Pain

Pain occurring in the wall of the chest is extremely common and may be due to pain in the muscles, ribs, and costo-chondral joints. A costo-chondral joint is formed at a point where the hard bone of the rib joins the softer bone (cartilage) that attaches to the breastbone. The costo-chondral joints frequently get an irritation termed a costo-chondritis. Pain can be localized to a small area the size of one or two fingertips and the area is tender to pressure. Sitting in a draft or exercise such as raking a lawn may aggravate the condition. Costo-chondritis is very common between the ages of thirty and sixty, and occasionally patients may become worried that it is the heart; the condition is much more common in women and occurs more often on the left side over the second and third costo-chondral joints. The pain is usually relieved by pain medications such as aspirin, but can recur over several months. The doctor may inject the joint with a combination of a local anesthetic and a cortisone compound, and this causes relief for several months, during which time nature heals the condition. The pain may return some time in the next few years. The important thing is to understand that it is a benign condition that never gets worse and does not lead to heart attacks or arthritis in other parts of the body. However, I must emphasize that in a few patients, costo-chondritis can coincide with heart pain.

## Arm Pain, Tingling, and Numbness

Many people experience tingling and numbness in the arm if the arm is rested over the back of a chair for several minutes or hours, or by sleeping on the arm in an unusual position. This pain is caused by pressure on the nerve, and normally subsides quickly once the unusual pressure has been removed. Arm pain, tingling, and numbness may occur when the nerves supplying the upper limb become involved by conditions such as arthritis of the spine in the neck region. Pressure is then exerted on the roots of the nerves as they emerge from the spine. Cervical disc disease is similar to the common condition, sciatica, which produces low back and leg pain. Pain arising from the above condition usually last several hours and may occur over many days. As well, it is an aching pain and is only occasionally associated with chest pain. Nerve and muscle pain does not get worse during vigorous walking. This serves to differentiate the pain from angina, which can cause pain in the arm during brisk walking. However, moderate to severe pain in the wrist or the arm occurring without any precipitating cause, especially if there is no tenderness on pressure or movement of the limb, warrants medical advice.

There are many other causes of chest pain, but because they are rare, they are not included in this discussion.

*Are age, sex, family history, and risk factors important in making a diagnosis of heart attack?*

Heart attack usually occurs in males over age thirty-five and in nonmenstruating females over age forty-eight. In recent years heart attacks have been observed in males age twenty-seven to thirty-four, but this occurrence is very rare. Such males usually have a very high blood cholesterol, hypertension, or rare diseases of the coronary arteries and a family history of heart attack before age fifty. Heart attacks occurring before age twenty-seven are extremely rare and may occur in patients with familial hypercholesterolemia who have a cholesterol in the range of 600 to 1,000 mg/deciliter (mg/dL). Menstruating females are often protected from heart attacks except those who smoke and simultaneously take the birth control pill, or in those with diabetes, hypertension, and rare familial hypercholesterolemia. The family history is important. Individuals with a strong family history, that is, a parent and one or more uncles or aunts dying of heart attacks before age fifty have an increased risk. These individuals should have a medical checkup, blood cholesterol, and HDL ("good") cholesterol measurements at about age twenty-five and have them repeated with a stress test at about age thirty.

The presence of risk factors such as a moderately high blood cholesterol, hypertension, or smoking do not assist in making the diagnosis. These risk factors indicate to the doctor only that the patient in the emergency room is at high risk for a heart attack.

# WHAT TO DO BEFORE THE AMBULANCE ARRIVES

I have given you the symptoms and signs of a heart attack so that you can quickly decide whether to go to an emergency room. Denial or wishful thinking that the pain will disappear in the next hour is about the worst thing you can do. Do not try to reach a physician for advice. Call the ambulance first, then you may make a call to your doctor or cardiologist. If you can't reach the doctor, leave a message; do not wait for a reply. If you are fortunate to live in an area where a mobile heart ambulance exists, then please use this service. If this is not available, use the ambulance service through the ambulance phone numbers or through the police or fire department. If no ambulances are available, use a taxi or have someone drive you immediately to the emergency room.

While waiting for the ambulance, which should arrive within minutes of your call, I can easily tell you, as would your spouse, to try to keep calm. However, very few can work up enough strength to stay calm in such a situation. Fear and panic causes further damage to the heart because they provoke the secretion of adrenaline, which increases the work of the heart and may increase the size of the heart attack or induce abnormal heart rhythms.

I offer the following advice to try and allay some of your anxiety. It is best to sit or lie propped up on three or four pillows and take a nitroglycerin tablet under the tongue. One tablet can do no harm. It will help calm your nerves as it will increase the blood supply to the coronary arteries. It also pools blood in the veins of the legs; therefore, less blood returns to the heart so there is less work for it to do. Nitroglycerin may decrease the size of a heart attack. It is reassuring to take one tablet under the tongue and believe that it will help. The drug is not as effective if you are lying flat. It is most effective if you sit up with your legs dangling over the edge of the bed or in a comfortable chair; this causes the blood to stay in the legs longer. Nitroglycerin may cause a headache, but this is to be expected because the drug dilates arteries including those in the scalp as well as the coronary arteries. There is no need to worry about the throbbing that you will feel in the head. The drug does not increase blood pressure.

All patients with coronary heart disease can benefit from having oxygen in the home for use in an emergency situation. You must break the vicious cycle of fear—and adrenaline. Oxygen given at this stage will certainly allay anxiety and panic. It is certainly helpful during the few minutes' wait. Put the oxygen mask right over your nose and mouth and breathe in the gas. There is nothing like believing that something will help when you are scared to death. I strongly recommend the use of oxygen and nitroglycerin as a technique to break the fear-anxiety-adrenaline reaction.

In treating life-threatening illnesses, a doctor must try to liberate the patient from fear and panic. The reassurance of the trusted physician or specialist and the use of morphine can be lifesaving. Until these are available, use the nitroglycerin and the oxygen. They will both help. Someone telling you to stay calm during the pain and fear of a heart attack is of no avail. Therefore, do the things that carry some hope. Remember, too, morphine is used not only to relieve pain but to relieve anxiety. Morphine is the best drug for this purpose, and you should not be opposed to its use. If a second injection is necessary even if your pain is mild, do not object to the physician's using a second or several doses of morphine.

Do not overdress. There is no reason to put on a vest, sweater, shirt, tie, jacket, or blouse that is difficult to remove. The garments will only have to be pulled off when you are in pain and lying on a stretcher in the emergency room. Therefore, if it is not excessively cold, do not put on a vest; use a pajama shirt or an open front blouse that can be easily opened to allow the doctor to examine you quickly and facilitate placement of the leads of the electrocardiogram (ECG, EKG) that must go on the chest. In addition, blood pressure is best taken with no garment around the arm. Every ambulance should have blankets to keep you warm. To reemphasize, it is a waste of precious time to try to remove clothing in the emergency room.

## MOBILE CORONARY CARE AMBULANCE

When a plaque of atheroma ruptures, a clot is formed within minutes. This causes centrally located chest pain associated with sweating and often shortness of breath. If you believe you are having a heart attack, quickly go to the emergency room of the nearest hospital. However, approximately 500,000 individuals with heart attacks die each year in the U.S. before reaching the hospital. The only way to save some of these lives is by the use of mobile heart squads. It is estimated that about 50,000 lives can be saved annually in North America by the use of heart squads. The first mobile coronary care ambulances were operated at the Royal Victoria Hospital in Belfast by Dr. J. F. Pantridge and Dr. J. S. Geddes[1] in 1965. The objective was to reach the patient quickly and stabilize the heart rhythm, relieve pain, as well as to afford reassurance and thus prevent death from abnormal heart rhythms. When the heart is found to be quivering and not contracting (ventricular fibrillation), the heart is defibrillated using a portable defibrillator. The success of such units led to the establishment of coronary care ambulances in Seattle and several other U.S. cities.[2]

During 1972, I tried to establish a mobile coronary care ambulance in Ottawa. Hospital approval to bypass the emergency room and take patients directly to the coronary care unit was achieved. However, after many months of stressful organizing and lobbying, the expected government grant support did not materialize. The government hoped at that time to give consideration to such projects during the early 1980s; however, I must emphasize that in the mid-1980s properly equipped emergency care ambulances are still lacking in Canada. Perhaps with the advent of the new drugs to dissolve clots in the coronary arteries and the emphasis on early administration of such treatment for success, special mobile units may become necessary if we wish to save the countless lives lost before reaching hospitals.

To reemphasize, in North America about half a million deaths occur outside the hospital whereas about 60,000 die from a heart attack in the hospital. It is estimated that coronary care units save about 30,000 to 40,000 lives annually in North America, at a very high but justifiable cost of running such units.

Importantly, it is simple to equip and run mobile emergency care units. The vital equipment consists of a lightweight portable defibrillator, an ECG recorder, intravenous preparations, morphine, and oxygen. A system in a city of 1 million people can be serviced by two units at a cost of about $100,000. It is the manpower that escalates the cost of running such units. It is feasible to send out a trained physician, a nurse, and a driver trained in cardiopulmonary resuscitation in such a unit. Perhaps doctors in training will see the need for such services in a community and help to organize systems with the help of their chiefs and with financial assistance from service clubs until government bodies are made aware of the life-saving potential that justifies the cost of mobile emergency care units.

I would hope that by 1990, the drugs to dissolve clots in the coronary artery may prove useful and safe to be given, intravenously, by trained staff running mobile heart squads.

It is distressing news that in the 1980s ambulances in the majority of cities in North America do not have portable defibrillators. Importantly, it is necessary to relieve the pain and fear that trigger abnormal heart rhythms that often lead to death. The ambulance attendant cannot give morphine. In addition, some ambulances do not have a springboard to allow chest massage.

The public can therefore assist by lobbying their member of parliament or congressional representative to achieve better mobile emergency care services. Visualize a heart attack victim, and consider, would it not be comforting to see a doctor, a nurse, and a trained driver at the bedside in the home within fifteen minutes of a call? The victim's pain and fear relieved and a life possibly saved! We can fly to the moon and perhaps build an artificial heart to save ten individuals, but alas, we cannot save millions for lack of a simple application of common sense.

North American and European hospitals offer coronary care facilities. These are specialized units where the staff and equipment can monitor the heart and where special intravenous drugs can be given to the heart. The hospital you choose should have the facilities necessary to dissolve clots in a coronary artery. If possible, choose a hospital that is well equipped and has a well-trained, experienced team who commonly perform:

- Coronary arteriography.
- Coronary angioplasty, i.e., the crushing of plaques of atheroma with a special balloon-tipped catheter.
- Cardiac surgery.

## WHAT PRECIPITATES OR CAUSES A HEART ATTACK?

The cause of a heart attack in the majority of cases is a blockage of a coronary artery by a blood clot. The clot usually occurs on the surface of a partially obstructing plaque of atheroma (see Chapter 1 and Figures 1-1, 1-4). The growth and enlargement of the atherosclerotic plaque are described in Chapter 1. The surface of a plaque ruptures and the plaque contains substances that increase the clotting of blood. A clot therefore forms on the surface of the rupture and also inside the plaque.

In the majority of patients with a heart attack, no precipitating factor can be identified. The individual may wonder, why today—what did I do wrong? Only occasionally is there some circumstantial evidence that may be related, for example, excessive unaccustomed exertion or severe stress. A large fatty meal, bedrest for several months, or overwork without undue distress do not appear to be precipitating factors. No one knows when a plaque of atheroma will rupture and cause a clot. If the blood is thicker and has a greater tendency to clot than normal, the individual is obviously at greater risk of having a heart attack. Some advice on how to prevent a blood clot is given in Chapter 8. Perhaps if we can't develop machines to tell us when a plaque of atheroma will rupture, we may get scientists to do further research to prevent formation of blood clots. Substances that cause clotting are liberated when the plaque ruptures; these substances are exposed to the flowing blood and a clot quickly forms, thus blocking the artery. Possibly, new drugs could be produced to inhibit the clotting substances present in the plaque. Importantly, I offer this hypothesis with the hope that a pharmaceutical firm or scientist will explore the possibility and produce a product that can prevent a fatal or nonfatal heart attack. Realistically, the situation will remain as it is for at least the next ten years.

# DRUGS TO DISSOLVE BLOOD CLOTS IN THE CORONARY ARTERY

Three drugs have been shown to be successful in dissolving clots in the coronary artery: streptokinase, urokinase, and tissue-type plasminogen activator (T-t plasminogen activator).

Streptokinase and urokinase have been shown to be useful when infused directly into the coronary artery, and they dissolve the clot in about 60 percent of patients. The drugs must be given within three hours of the onset of symptoms to be successful, and some benefit is seen in up to four hours. Streptokinase given through an arm vein (IV) only has a 40 percent chance of dissolving a clot in the coronary artery. The discovery of T-t plasminogen activator will render IV streptokinase obsolete. The new and major advance is the use of tissue-type plasminogen activator. This drug is more successful and does not cause allergic reactions as seen occasionally with streptokinase.[3] Clinical trials done in 1984 and 1985 have documented the success of this drug when it is given intravenously. Randomized clinical trials are in progress to document that this dissolution of clot results in a stronger heart muscle and saves lives. Widespread use of this drug is expected by 1987. Thus, there is great hope for patients who have suffered a heart attack, provided they can get quickly to the emergency room of an appropriate hospital.

In some patients, after the clot is dissolved, it may be necessary to crush the underlying plaque of atheroma with a special balloon catheter (angioplasty), as discussed in Chapter 11.

# WHAT TO EXPECT IN THE HOSPITAL

If you still have pain on arrival at the emergency room, you can be reassured that the pain will be relieved within five minutes. Usually no time is wasted. The emergency room staff are primed to move quickly to deal with ambulance cases, in particular, those suspected to be heart attack victims. Thus, while your friend or your spouse gives your particulars, you are mainly expected to say to the nurse or the doctor that you are having chest pain. Point to the area of pain, indicating that it is severe or very severe and that you are scared and would like something as soon as possible for the pain. You can then cooperate by answering all the other questions that the doctor may wish to ask. You will usually have to state whether you are allergic to medications. You will quickly receive an intravenous injection of morphine, which relieves the pain in two to five minutes. Since the injection is given intravenously, very small doses are used; for example, it may be given in 2 mg increments every minute until the pain is completely relieved. Remember, do not be embarrassed to say that you are scared. A heart attack makes everyone afraid and the doctor may sometimes forget this. Intramuscular injections are avoided since the needle damages muscle cells, which then release an enzyme, creatinine kinase, similar to that released from the damaged heart muscle and may cause confusion in the diagnosis. You are quickly hooked up to continuous oxygen, and a blood pressure cuff is placed around your arm.

The doctor examines you and asks you relevant questions. There is very little reason for the doctor to ask more than 12 questions, since the diagnosis is usually easily made from your description of the chest pain and from the electrocardiogram that is done within minutes of your arrival. The electrocardiogram is called an ECG or EKG. *Electro-* means "electrical," *cardio-* means "heart," and *-gram* means "writing." The ECG writes the electrical rhythm and rate of each heartbeat. You are immediately hooked up to a cardiac monitor; small electrodes are placed on your chest similar to the ECG electrodes and these are connected to the monitor. The electrodes detect the electrical impulses from the heart, which are recorded continuously on a monitored screen. The nurses and doctors can see the visual display of the continuous electrocardiogram, showing each heartbeat with the important heart rate and rhythm of the heart.

It seems reasonable at this stage for you to understand what is meant by the rhythm of the heart. The rhythm is normally regular, that is, each beat comes regularly with the same interval between beats. In other words, the rhythm is as regular as the beat of a clock. If the rhythm becomes very irregular, it can be easily observed from the monitor and it may require treatment. The commonest reason for an irregular rhythm is extra beats (premature beats). Such beats are often found in normal people, but often increase during a heart attack as the area of damaged muscle causes electrical disturbances and fires extra discharges that interrupt the normal clocklike rhythm. If these extra beats are frequent or of a special variety, they act as warning signals and the doctor suppresses these beats by giving a drug called lidocaine intravenously and then through a continuous intravenous drip. The drug is very effective in stabilizing the heart rhythm and has no serious side effects, so you have no need to worry or be afraid. In some hospitals, as soon as the diagnosis of heart attack is made, the drug lidocaine is given routinely to all patients and continued for one to two days.

I intend to give you reassuring news. It is important for you to start seeing the brighter side of things. Once the morphine is given, the worst is over. You are out of danger since you have made it to the hospital, where expert care is available. Most deaths occur before the patient reaches the hospital. Those who die before reaching the hospital have either a very large heart attack, experience electrical disturbances that cause the heart to quiver (ventricular fibrillation) or stop beating, or have remained too long outside of the hospital with extensive damage to the heart muscle.

Blood is taken and several blood tests are done; the ones that are necessary for the diagnosis are those for cardiac enzymes. The heart muscle cells that are deprived of blood undergo a series of changes ranging from injury to death of the cells and liberate three of these enzymes, which can be detected in the blood; the most reliable is the creatine kinase (CK). In some hospitals, the special fraction of CK (CK-MB) that is derived solely from heart muscle is measured to distinguish it from the release from ordinary skeletal muscle.

From here on I believe that the less you know, the better it is for you. The damaged heart muscle will heal itself over the next few weeks. It is pointless to start inquiring about what artery, how big a heart attack, or what are my chances, Doc? You will have enough time to inquire about the details later, and this is best done about one week after the heart attack. The muscle will be healing and you will be able to stand the news.

There is no reason to be brave, and feel that you must know and can hear the bad news. More bad news brings more alarm to your system, which pours out more of the dangerous adrenaline and worsens the damaged muscle, or produces abnormal heart rhythms. I draw your attention to Figures 6-1 and 6-2, the heart under stress. All you need to know is that you have or have not sustained a heart attack. If you have a heart attack, you need rest and reassurance; let others do the worrying.

## Coronary Care Unit (CCU)

The patient is moved fairly quickly from the emergency room to the CCU. This can take one to four hours depending on the hospital bed space. Hospitals that render efficient heart care strive to get patients to the CCU within a half to one hour of emergency room arrival. The CCU is a special area of the hospital, usually four to ten beds with a staff of specially trained doctors and nurses along with sophisticated electronic equipment to deal with heart attack patients. It will take some adjustment, over six to twenty-four hours, for a patient to get used to all the gadgets. The patient will have already had an electrocardiogram in the emergency room, and this is repeated in the CCU and once daily for three days. The patient is attached to a cardiac monitor similar to the one used in the emergency room.

The electrocardiogram is the main diagnostic tool and can accurately make the diagnosis in the majority of patients. In more than 95 percent of the cases during a first heart attack, typical findings occur on the electrocardiogram and are easily recognized. If the first ECG is only suggestive of a heart attack, the repeat ECG six and twenty-four hours later usually gives an accurate diagnosis. In patients with a previous heart attack, the electrocardiogram is less diagnostic and is positive in about 75 percent of the cases. To reemphasize, less than 10 percent of patients during the first heart attack have an electrocardiogram that may not be diagnostic and it can be normal in about 5 percent of the cases. However, when the ECG is repeated six to twenty-four hours later, typical changes confirm the diagnosis of a heart attack. It is necessary in a difficult case for the doctor in the emergency room to pay special attention to the patient's description of the chest discomfort. Therefore, in such cases, the patient must put up with answering several questions posed by several doctors from junior to chief. Perhaps the fortunate patient does not have a heart attack. In this case, the doctor may elect to admit the individual for observation for twenty-four to forty-eight hours. The creatine kinase (CK), a cardiac enzyme, starts to increase about four to six hours after the heart attack and may be normal in some cases if tested for very early during the attack. A careful physician often repeats the ECG and blood test for CK about six hours after the patient arrives in the emergency room. If both ECG and CK are normal and the description of chest pain is not suggestive of a heart attack, the doctor may elect to send the individual home. The patient is advised to return to the emergency room if the pain recurs. A risk is therefore taken and the public must understand that the doctor may not be able to admit every patient and that the pain may be due to other causes. Policy varies depending on the physician in charge. If doubt exists, the patient is admitted and if three ECGs done over a forty-eight-hour period and repeat cardiac enzymes are normal, then a heart attack can be excluded with confidence. In very rare instances, the diagnosis is firmly established only on the third or fourth day of the illness.

A routine chest X-ray is given. It cannot diagnose a heart attack; however, it is very useful in making the diagnosis of heart failure. A heart attack causes weakness of a segment of the heart muscle of the left ventricle. Therefore, the heart does not contract as strongly as before. The left ventricle may not be able to eject most of the blood delivered to it from the right side of the heart via the lung. Therefore some blood builds up and stays longer in the lungs because the right side of the heart is normal and keeps pumping blood into the lungs and into the left ventricle. The excess blood in the lungs causes a leakage of fluid into and around air sacs and forms water (edema) in the lungs. This lung (pulmonary) edema shows up on the chest X-ray and is easy for the doctor to recognize as heart failure. Heart failure causes shortness of breath and is quickly relieved by oxygen, morphine, and a patch of nitroglycerin paste or ointment, which is applied to the skin. The drug, furosemide, removes salt and water from the lungs and body through the kidney and is very effective in producing relief in patients with pulmonary edema. Therefore, if you get short of breath, you should inform the nurse so that effective treatment may be given. Other medications are available for managing severe heart failure; however, the majority of cases respond to treatment with furosemide, oxygen, morphine, and nitropaste.

Occasionally the blood pressure is very low and drug combinations are given intravenously to maintain the systolic blood pressure between 90 and 100 mm Hg. Blood pressure of 95 to 105 systolic is very common in patients with heart attacks but it can be 110 to 140 in those who had slightly higher blood pressure before the heart attack.

In some units, other instruments are used to monitor the amount of blood ejected from the left ventricle, that is, the cardiac output. Because of the many parameters that are measured, several veins in the arm may be used for the introduction of a venous tube, which is usually about one to two inches long and is not harmful.

Nuclear scans can be helpful in the few patients who do not have classical diagnostic findings on the electrocardiogram or cardiac enzymes. It is not routine to have nuclear scans because the ECG and blood test for cardiac enzymes are sufficient in more than 90 percent of the cases for a firm diagnosis. Several tests increase the cost to both patient and state.

A monitoring catheter may be inserted into the right heart to monitor the pressure within the heart; this helps to make the diagnosis of heart failure, and assists with evaluation of the treatment in critically ill patients.

The procedure for introducing the catheter is relatively simple. The skin area over the vein is infiltrated with local anesthetic. The specially made fine tube (catheter) has a tiny balloon and sensing devices at its tip. The catheter is inserted into the vein and threaded into the right ventricle and the pulmonary artery. The position is verified by X-ray.

Patients with severe heart failure and very low blood pressure may require several drugs and fluid replacement given intravenously. The monitoring catheter that is positioned in the pulmonary artery is very useful for the infusion of intravenous preparations.

*Day One.* In hospitals where facilities exist, special drugs that dissolve clots are given within one to two hours of arrival in the emergency room, or the CCU once the diagnosis of a heart attack is established.

Treatment is continued with oxygen, which can be discontinued after twenty-four hours in the majority of patients. The amount of oxygen in the arterial blood is tested by a simple measurement, and if this is normal, the oxygen is usually discontinued, which is reassuring news.

Generally, no food or drink is allowed for the first eight hours, since the process of digestion steals blood from the heart; also if vomiting occurs, vomitus may be aspirated into the lung.

During the stay in the coronary care unit, the patient receives sufficient sedation, mainly with oxazepam, to prevent anxiety and to ensure adequate rest.

I emphasize that during the first eight hours reassurance is crucial. The patient must be reassured that the worst is over since the majority of deaths occur before admission to hospital. This reassurance can be given by the medical resident staff and nurses, but must be reinforced by the physician in charge, since his or her authority is very persuasive in relieving the fear and anxiety.

*Day Two.* A light diet is usually given and increased over a few days to a normal diet. On the second day, patients are usually sitting at the bedside.

*Days Three to Five.* Late on the second or on the third day, the patient is moved from the coronary care unit to an intermediate care area or to a ward with other patients. In the standard room, the patient is allowed more freedom each day starting with walks to the bathroom and progressing then by day five to walks in the corridor of the hospital. If the individual is making a good recovery, the intravenous tubes are removed by the third or fourth day. The education process will now begin and both husband and wife are usually given instructions together in a question and answer period each day. The individual is often concerned that pain is no longer present and wonders why it is necessary to stay in the hospital. The pain of a heart attack usually disappears between one and six hours, and in most patients, there is usually no recurrence of pain during the hospital stay and in many there is no pain for several years. By the fourth day, the patient is very well and enjoys meals and walks around alone. At this stage the doctor will wish to discuss the question of how much rest is necessary. The patient must understand that a blockage of a coronary artery has taken place. This caused damage and death to a segment of heart muscle cells. Special cells in the body that form bridges (scar tissue cells) move into the area and form scar tissue joining the two normal areas of heart muscle. The scar tissue is similar to that following the healing of a surgical incision. It takes time for scar tissue to form and heal. The healing process usually takes three to six weeks. During the 1950s and 1960s it was common practice to keep patients in hospital for four to eight weeks. However, in the 1970s it became apparent that after seven days, if there were no complications, most patients could be allowed home.

In most hospitals, patients are discharged home between the seventh and fourteenth day depending on the size of infarction, complications, and their home situation.

*Day Six.* By the sixth day, the patient is walking approximately 100 feet, 2 or 3 times daily, and by the seventh to the tenth day, has been supervised while walking up one flight of stairs and may have had a stroll on the treadmill to reach a heart rate of 120 per minute. The heart rhythm is usually checked for twenty-four hours to ensure that severe rhythm disturbances do not occur.

## EMOTIONAL IMPACT OF A HEART ATTACK

Most patients undergo a traumatic mental experience. Uncertainty about the financial impact, the work situation, relationships, and in particular, sexual activity may cause depression and anxiety. Social workers, nurses, and the medical team must find time to listen and talk to the patient. Explanations and answers must be clear so that the patient understands that, after a heart attack, a normal life is possible for the majority. The sophisticated gadgets of modern medicine cannot replace the reassuring words of an understanding caring physician.

Reassurance is important not only to the patient but also to the patient's family. The patient's relative is often in distress and must receive adequate counseling from the nursing staff, medical health staff, and the physician in charge. During the entire hospital stay, a few minutes spent each day with the relative to answer questions is most rewarding and greatly appreciated.

## Depression and Anxiety

The majority of heart attack patients experience some degree of depression and anxiety. To combat this complication, both the doctor and the nurses must communicate with the patient in an open and frank manner so that the patient can ventilate and have all questions answered during his or her last seven days in the hospital. A social worker may have to be involved in some cases; supportive home visits, advice on job orientation, and discussions regarding financial matters may be necessary. Discussions are necessary during the next three months; two weekly visits to an understanding family doctor may help to dissipate depression with the recognition that all is not lost. The individual must understand that this depression and anxiety with the associated weakness and tiredness are normal and will be alleviated with time. It takes six weeks for the damaged muscle to heal and form a firm scar. During the same six weeks, the anxiety and depression dissipate in the majority. The heart attack patient must understand that it is mainly the first four weeks that will be tough. Thereafter, the assistance of an exercise program, the ability to drive again, and the return of sexual activity help to remove despair. Time heals all wounds including the muscle damage and psychological insults. A few (about 1 percent of patients) require antidepressant drugs. They are nonaddicting and can be very useful when given as a single bedtime dose for three to a maximum of twelve weeks. An exercise rehabilitation program is very useful in many respects and is of definite assistance in the management of most heart attack patients.

# RETURN TO WORK

Most patients under age sixty are advised to return to work between six and eight weeks after discharge. The return date should take into account the patient's age, financial resources, existing diseases, and type of work. The physical and emotional stress associated with the job should be thoroughly explored.


# ADVICE ON DIET

Patients over age sixty are not given strict diet prescriptions since there is no scientific evidence that such diets are of any value in prevention. Those who are overweight should be encouraged to follow a reduction diet, but control of elevated blood cholesterol by diet in this age group is not rewarding. A low-salt diet is prescribed for patients with heart failure who require water pills (diuretics) or the heart pill, digoxin, as well as for the previously hypertensive patient. Patients less than age sixty are advised on the use of a weight reduction diet and a modified diet to reduce cholesterol and saturated fat intake (see Chapter 2). Lipid-lowering drugs are not prescribed but may be considered for patients who have cholesterol levels greater than 250 mg/dL. In patients less than age sixty, the serum cholesterol and high-density lipoprotein ("good") cholesterol are estimated for the patient in the hospital. The estimation is done mainly for future hospital reference and to reassure the patient who may be fearful of an elevated cholesterol. Some patients may inquire about their HDL cholesterol level, and the doctor usually carries out a blood cholesterol test in the hospital and another about three months later. Alcohol should be avoided for the first four weeks; thereafter one to two ounces daily are allowed, mainly because of the sedative effect. Alcohol is restricted if heart failure is present or if the heart is enlarged.

# EXERCISE AND REHABILITATION

Patients with uncomplicated myocardial infarctions are advised to increase activity so as to return to about 90 percent of the preinfarction level in three months. Types of exercise are discussed in detail in Chapter 5. Exercise at home is graduated as follows: During the first three days at home, walk in the house; for the remainder of the first week, walk outside the home 50 to 100 yards daily. The second week, walk 200 yards once or twice daily. The third week, cover 300 yards once or twice daily. The fourth week, go a quarter mile or 440 yards once or twice daily. During the fifth week, walk a half mile daily, and during the sixth week, one mile once or twice daily. This is a rough estimate of what you should be doing during the weeks after a heart attack. Thereafter, if you feel well and have no chest pain, you should be able to do much more exercise; this includes joining exercise programs. One- to three-mile walks are usual by the eighth week. Doubles tennis, golf, and similar past times are reasonable at three months.

Patients may join supervised exercise programs provided there is no evidence of:

1.   Heart failure.
2.   Enlargement of the heart.
3.   Angina.
4.   Abnormal heart rhythm such as frequent extra beats.
5.   Moderate to severe problems with heart valves.

A stress test is useful at some point, especially if the individual is inquiring about further activities. In patients under age sixty a stress test done after the twelfth week should result in the patient being able to do six to nine minutes of walking on the treadmill. Patients who can complete about nine minutes without undue shortness of breath, chest pain, or ECG changes, which are indicative of oxygen lack to the heart muscle, are usually allowed to engage in all exercise activities. However, competitive squash and extreme exertion should be avoided. Patients who can complete six minutes, but need to stop because of fatigue, tiredness, or leg discomfort and who show a normal heart rate and blood pressure without showing an abnormal heart rhythm or ECG changes, are allowed to participate in a restricted and, if possible, supervised exercise program, but they should be retested in three months. Exercise programs should be individualized. There are many useful rehabilitation programs attached to major hospitals. Provided that adequate supervision is obtained, exercise programs play a great role in assisting patients to maintain good body tone and to return to participation in games, sexual activity, and work, which they were accustomed to before a heart attack. I strongly endorse exercise programs, provided that the patient is stress-tested and conditions that contraindicate exercise programs are reviewed by the physician for each individual. The patient should be informed that there is no evidence that moderate to strenuous exercise prevents heart attacks or limits the size of a heart attack. The physician should recognize the minority of patients in whom a very gradual program or only mild exercises are appropriate. Walking certainly provides safe and adequate exercise.

Because you have had a heart attack, it does not mean that you will be crippled for life. About 10 million North Americans can testify that you can recover from a heart attack and go on to live a very active and normal life. The majority return to the same job. Within three to six months, the majority engage in the same activities as prior to the heart attack. Tennis, golf, and skiing are only a few of the many activities that are enjoyed. Some individuals lead a more active life and learn to handle stress and often report that they feel better than ten years prior to their heart attack. If you like jogging, you should know that six months after their heart attack, more than 60 percent of patients are able to jog one to three miles daily. I am not suggesting that you do this, but if you enjoy jogging, then one to two miles four times weekly will improve your endurance. Similar exercises including a one- to three-mile walk and stair climbing are suitable activities.

## Don'ts

1.  Do not do static exercises such as weightlifting or push-ups. Such exercise uses sustained muscular con-

traction that squeezes the blood vessels, and thus increases blood pressure and the work of the heart.

2. Do not exercise immediately after a meal. Wait one to two hours after a light snack or two to three hours after a heavy meal. Do not exercise if you have a fever.

3. Do not stop exercising suddenly; always warm up and cool down for five to ten minutes.

4. During the first six weeks at home, do not engage in strenuous exercise or housework such as heavy cleaning or repairs, gardening such as raking leaves or mowing the lawn, or snow shoveling.

5. Do not take a hot or cold shower immediately before or after exercise. Do not take a sauna because the heat dilates the vessels in the skin and steals blood away from the heart and the brain.

## RETIREMENT

It is important to recognize that retirement may well be a problem for many individuals, especially those who do not have enough hobbies to keep them sufficiently occupied. They become bored and depressed, and therefore retirement must be selective. It is necessary to try to have all patients get back to work since this prevents the development of neurosis and depression. However, there is no doubt that returning to a job that was previously distressing to the individual can lead to further harm. Patients who can afford to change jobs or retire and have enough hobbies do extremely well. The good news is that the disease may burn itself out. A new, less distressing lifestyle may halt the progression of coronary heart disease, and individuals who are informed that they have serious complications and cannot participate in exercise programs often live for more than ten years. Individuals who have had large heart attacks or have complications that restrict exercise programs are strongly advised to retire, especially if they are over sixty.

## SMOKING

Patients under age sixty-five are strongly advised to discontinue smoking completely since there is evidence that this does prevent further heart attacks. Individuals who find it a major problem to quit smoking are advised to try a pipe, since pipe smoking does not appear to increase the risk of heart attacks. Individuals who give up smoking may gain weight, and it is necessary for them to have adequate dietary counseling as well as maintenance on an exercise program. Many drugs used to treat angina or high blood pressure do not work in smokers. (The dangers of smoking are outlined in Chapter 4.)

## SEXUAL ACTIVITIES

Sex is a part of living. For the majority, it is one of the most enjoyable, satisfying, stress-relieving activities that life provides. Most of what is said relates to men because the heart attack rate is far more common in men than women. Also, men have far more hang-ups about sex than women, especially since a man cannot will an erection. Fear interferes with performance; thus some men, owing to a lack of proper discussion with their doctor before hospital discharge, develop fears that may cause problems with sexual function. In addition, the female partner develops fear and apprehension that intercourse could cause the death of her husband. The female partner may therefore turn the whole thing off. This disturbance in a marital relationship can be quite traumatic and increase the anxiety and depression that is so common after a heart attack.

It is important for males to understand that a heart attack does not cause impotence, and that if you do not have intercourse for three to six weeks, it will not alter sexual performance in the future. The good news is that six to twelve weeks after a heart attack, more than 85 percent of patients are able to engage in sexual intercourse with the same frequency as before. To reemphasize, a heart attack is not the end of your sex life. Some physicians believe that sex can be resumed about one week after discharge from the hospital. But the majority of physicians agree that it is reasonable and safe to resume intercourse about six to eight weeks after a heart attack. There is no hard-and-fast rule; you should do what comes naturally and without fear. If, about three weeks after discharge, you are able to walk one mile and climb two flights of stairs without chest discomfort or undue shortness of breath and experience the urge to have sex with your usual partner, then you should go ahead without fear of precipitating another heart attack.

The amount of physical exertion required during sexual intercourse is equivalent to walking up about three flights of stairs or a brisk one-mile walk. Most heart attack patients should be engaging in this type of exercise about six weeks after a heart attack. If during such activity there is no chest discomfort or undue shortness of breath, sexual activities are considered safe. In a study of 6,000 cases of sudden death, only thirty-four were related to sexual intercourse and twenty-seven of those deaths occurred during extramarital sexual relations. Sudden death or heart attack is extremely rare when the heart attack patient engages in intercourse with the usual partner. Most deaths in males during intercourse occur while engaging with partners other than their wives. Middle-aged males who have been married for a number of years are at greatest risk. Intercourse with a much younger extramarital female partner may lead to more emotional reactions, causing a much higher increase of blood pressure and heart rate, thus putting the heart under severe strain. Furthermore, such a relation may also be accompanied by the ingestion of a large meal and alcohol, which adds to cardiac work.

It is advisable to use the position with which you are most accustomed. There is no reason to change to side to side or female on top if this was not the most often practiced and most favorable position. If the patient is male and erection is easily achieved, the female on top—superior crouched—is often recommended. In this position, the woman has both knees touching the bed for traction. Therefore she is the active partner. However, what is most familiar is always the best position as it increases confidence in the male and allays anxiety in the female, who is afraid that the husband may die or have a heart attack during intercourse. Importantly, studies show that blood pressure and heart rate are not significantly affected by whether the male is on top or the female is on top.

There is no need to decrease the frequency of sexual activity. To reemphasize, after three months if there is no chest pain, undue shortness of breath or palpitations on walking two to three miles or climbing three to four flights of stairs or jogging one mile, the individual should be capable of enjoying the same sexual frequency, style, and intensity as before the heart attack.

## Don'ts

These apply to the first three months after a heart attack and for patients with chest pain on effort (angina) or heart failure.

1.  Do not take a hot shower immediately before intercourse. Hot showers or saunas dilate vessels of the skin, thus stealing blood from the heart and the brain.
2.  Do not have intercourse immediately after a heavy meal; wait two to three hours.
3.  Do not have more than one drink of alcohol or beer and indulge in intercourse. More than three drinks consumed in two hours will make it more difficult to achieve an erection and may also decrease heart muscle contraction.
4.  Do not engage in extramarital intercourse or relationships with an unusual pattern.
5.  Smoking can also decrease sexual performance (see Chapter 4).

## Suggestions

1.  A simple exercise program improves physical endurance and nearly always increases sexual performance. Therefore, start your walking program one week after discharge and increase it to a brisk one to two miles walk daily by the sixth week. Each week increase from

one, then two, then three flights of stairs by the sixth week. If your hospital or community offers a rehabilitation program, it is wise to join this with the advice of your cardiologist. Or plan your own program with some common sense (see Chapter 5). At this stage, you should know how to take your pulse and try to keep the heart rate for about five minutes within the target zone, i.e., 60 to 70 percent of your maximal heart rate (Table 5-1). After a few months of exercise, if you feel well, you can keep the heart rate in the target zone for about five to ten minutes during thirty minutes of exercise. A stress test at this stage may increase your confidence, and your physician can advise on additional exercises.

2. Rest is more important before rather than after sexual activity, although if you feel tired after the activity and feel like sleeping, certainly it is wise to have a half- to one-hour rest. Therefore, if possible, have intercourse in the morning after a night of sleep or any other time after having a half- to one-hour rest or relaxation.

3. If you are very short of breath or develop chest discomfort during intercourse, stop and take nitroglycerin. Importantly, discomfort during your first sexual relations does not mean the discomfort may occur again. It does not indicate that you are likely to develop a heart attack during intercourse. However, if pain does occur again or if there is any difficulty with sexual activity, be sure to discuss this with your doctor at the next office visit, which is usually about six weeks after discharge. Medications given on discharge may interfere with sexual performance and these may be reduced at your next office visit. In particular, diuretics (water pills) and less commonly beta-blockers, antihypertensive drugs, or antidepressants can alter sexual performance. However, patients who have angina and get pain on intercourse can get relief with beta-blockers, nifedipine, or other anti-anginal drugs.

## DO YOU NEED A BETA-BLOCKER?

Beta-blocking drugs are discussed in Chapter 9, and the present discussion explains mainly the rationale for their use in patients after a heart attack. Beta-blockers block the action of adrenaline and noradrenaline at receptor sites on the surface of cells. They cause a reduction in heart rate; therefore, less oxygen is required by the weakened heart muscle. They decrease the force of contraction of the heart muscles, and this further decreases the work and the amount of oxygen required by the heart. Most of the effects on the heart and arteries are related to this block of the actions of stress hormones. Beta-blockers stabilize the heart rhythm and can prevent extra beats, in particular, those that are precipitated by mental and physical stress. They can prevent some episodes of ventricular fibrillation, which is the cause of sudden death.

I must reemphasize that beta-blockers are the only drugs that are proven by studies to prevent death from heart attacks.[5, 6] When given to patients from about the seventh day after a heart attack and for two years, they significantly reduce the incidence of death from heart attack including sudden death.[5] They also reduce the recurrent rate of subsequent heart attacks. About 70 of every 100 heart patients are eligible for treatment with beta-blockers and these include patients who have angina after the heart attack.

In the United Kingdom, a survey of actively practicing British consulting cardiologists was carried out during 1984 to determine their practices when prescribing beta-blockers after a heart attack. Half of the cardiologists reported that they use beta-blockers in all patients who can take the drug starting about one week after the heart attack and the drug is given for about two years. The other half reported that they gave the beta-blockers to patients at high risk.[7] I strongly recommend a beta-blocker to all post–heart attack patients from day seven if there is no contraindication to their use.

Despite the beneficial effects of beta-blockers, about 30 percent of the physicians in North America are reluctant to prescribe the drugs for patients after a heart attack. This reluctance stems from the teaching of a minority of experts. The argument of the physicians who oppose the routine use of beta-blockers is as follows: Although the beta-blocker, timolol, has been shown to cause a 33 percent reduction in cardiac deaths in a well-run multicenter randomized clinical trial,[5] a 33 percent reduction means that of every 100 patients with a heart attack treated with a beta-blocker, "only" 3 lives can be saved. That is, if you take 100 heart attack patients discharged from hospital, studies have established that 10 patients will die in the next year; 33 percent of the 10 deaths can be saved—3 patients. Thus these physicians believe that it is not worthwhile to treat 100 patients with a beta-blocker to save "only" 3. Some physicians use expensive, sophisticated tests to define high-risk patients who are likely to die in the next year. Beta-blockers are then given to the few patients who are termed high-risk. However, prediction by tests, especially stress tests, nuclear scans, and Holter monitoring can be misleading.

To these opposing physicians, I pose the following question: The next twenty years of extensive and expensive research may produce a medication capable of a 60 percent reduction in deaths in patients who have had a heart attack and then treated for one year. This result will be accepted by all physicians as good news. If the majority of physicians will then agree to treat 100 to save 6, why not treat 100 to save 3 at present? Is the difference between 6 and 3 that great?

The dose of a beta-blocker used for the prevention of death and recurrent heart attacks is not high and side effects are infrequent. A fall in pulse rate from the usual average 70 per minute to 55 per minute is expected if the drug is working. On mild to moderate exercise the heart rate stays under 120 per minute as opposed to racing to 140 to 150 with a single moderate amount of exercise. The slowing of the pulse is a good effect; therefore, do not be afraid of a heart rate of 50 to 60 per minute. Only a few patients, less than 10 percent, get symptoms of dizziness if the pulse falls below 50 per minute. The dose of drug is then reduced by half and the pulse stabilizes between 54 and 64 per minute. In a few patients, the drug has to be discontinued because too much slowing may occur on a very small dose. Fortunately these sensitive patients are rare (1 percent).

The commonly used beta-blocking drugs are:

1. Timolol: 5 mg twice daily for one week then 10 mg twice daily.

2. Propranolol: 40 mg twice daily for two weeks then 80 mg twice daily for one month followed by 160 to 240 mg long-acting once daily.
3. Nadolol: 40 mg daily for one week then 80 to a maximum of 120 mg daily.
4. Metoprolol: 50 mg twice daily for two weeks then 100 mg twice daily.

Many other beta-blockers are available, but the ones listed have been shown to be useful in post–heart attack patients. Propranolol and metoprolol may not confer cardiac protection in smokers. Therefore it is important to also discontinue smoking.

If you notice any side effects, especially wheezing, increased shortness of breath, dizziness, or impotence, reduce the daily dose by half and consult your doctor. Impotence is very rare but does occur. The incidence is about 4 in every 100 patients treated. As emphasized, heart attacks do not cause impotence but can decrease sexual activity; therefore it may not be the drug. In any event, alteration in sexual activity should prompt the doctor to reduce the dose of beta-blocking drugs. If there is no improvement, the drug may be discontinued. The effect on sexual function is quickly reversible. If you are taking water pills (diuretics), they cause a higher incidence of sexual dysfunction than beta-blockers.

The use of beta-blocking drugs can save between 15,000 and 20,000 lives annually in the United States and, as well, many nonfatal heart attacks can be prevented.

## PACEMAKERS

A cardiac pacemaker is an electronic device that delivers electrical stimuli to the heart. It may be necessary to insert a temporary pacemaker in a few patients in whom the heart attack has disturbed the electrical conducting system of the heart.

In about 2 in every 100 patients with a heart attack, the sinus node pacemaker in the right atrium and the electrical pathway connecting the atrium and the ventricle become damaged and the heart rate becomes very slow (see Figure 15-1). The heart rate may fall to less than thirty-six beats per minute. If the condition does not respond to drugs such as atropine, a temporary pacemaker, which is required only for two to five days, is inserted through a vein.

The procedure is a simple one. The temporary pacemaker consists of a pacing wire that is inserted through a vein in the neck, usually the subclavian vein. The skin over the vein is infiltrated with a local anesthetic so that the procedure is not painful. A pacing catheter is threaded through the vein to reach the inside of the right ventricle. The passage of the pacing catheter is usually done under fluoroscopic (X-ray) control since the wire is radio-opaque and can be seen on the X-ray. Occasionally the procedure is done with the assistance of the electrocardiogram and the final position of the catheter verified by X-ray. The external end of the wire catheter is connected to a battery-operated pulse generator. The pulse generator is set, for example, at about sixty-five beats per minute, and commences pacing if the heartbeat falls below this set rate. The pacemaker works (fires) only when it is required, that is, on demand. Complications are very few for the insertion and maintenance of the pacemaker in the heart for two to seven days.

## Permanent Pacemaker

Approximately 1 million people across the globe have permanent pacemakers (.5 million in the United States). A pacemaker is often required in the management of patients who have complete heart block or a condition called sick sinus syndrome, which I will discuss shortly.

In about 1 in every 200 patients with a heart attack, the electrical conducting system is permanently damaged. The heart rate becomes very slow, less than 36 per minute, and loss of consciousness may occur. The condition is called heart block because there is a block of the conduction of electrical impulses from the atrium through the main electrical tunnel (atrioventricular node) that transmits the impulses to the ventricle (Figure 15-1). The atrium normally contracts at seventy-two beats per minute and in heart block continues to beat at seventy-two per minute but the ventricles fail to receive the message to do the same. Pacemaker cells in the ventricle may create an electrical impulse but beat at a rate less than thirty-six per minute. Occasionally, in this condition, the ventricles fail to contract, as there is no electrical stimulus, or the ventricle quivers (ventricular fibrillation) and loss of consciousness occurs. In such patients a pacemaker site in the ventricle may suddenly restart the heart and the patient recovers in a few seconds. A similar condition occurs in individuals who have a rare degenerative disease of the conduction system, simply, the electrical wires of the heart are bad, but the heart muscle, coronary arteries, and the valves are relatively normal. Cases of heart block may also occur in childhood because of congenital defect in the conduction system, but fortunately the condition is rare. In patients with degenerative disease of the conduction system and with congenital heart block, the remainder of the heart is completely normal and the insertion of a permanent pacemaker allows for normal activity and lifespan.

As mentioned above, a permanent pacemaker may also be necessary in patients who have a condition called sick sinus syndrome. In this condition, because of coronary heart disease, the normal sinus node pacemaker may have been destroyed because of lack of blood supply. The heart beat then becomes erratic; at times, the heart may beat very slowly (36 to 48 per minute) and at other times beats quickly (100 to 150 per minute). The patient may complain of dizziness or transient loss of consciousness (syncope). A permanent pacemaker is inserted and the patient gets complete relief of symptoms if the symptoms were due to a sick sinus node. The condition is rare and is most often seen in individuals over age sixty-five. It is important to document that these symptoms are due to a sick sinus because they can also be caused by several other conditions, including lack of circulation to the brain, that a pacemaker will not help.

### What a Pacemaker Will Not Do

1. A pacemaker does not cause the heart muscle to contract more forcefully; therefore, it does not help heart failure except in some cases where a very slow heart rate was contributing to the heart failure.

2. It does not increase the blood supply through the coronary arteries; therefore, it does not help chest pain or angina or prevent a heart attack.

3. A pacemaker does not replace the usual cardiac medications prescribed for various heart conditions. You need to take the medications prescribed by your doctor for heart failure, angina, or other conditions that may exist.

A pacemaker is a great device but it does only what it is designed to do. It stimulates the electrical system of the heart so that the heart beats at the correct time and at an appropriate rate. A pacemaker can prolong life provided the problem is that of too slow a heart rate or no heartbeat because of heart block.

## Types of Pacemakers

There are numerous pacemaker systems on the market. Your cardiologist or cardiac surgeon will choose the one appropriate for you. Usually, the individual requiring a pacemaker is admitted to the hospital. The pacemaker is inserted by a cardiac surgeon and occasionally by a cardiologist during a simple operation. A pacemaker consists of a heart generator that weighs about forty grams and is implanted under the skin of the lower abdomen or near the collarbone. The tips (leads) of the pacing wire that emerge from the pacemaker generator are inserted into the vein and threaded through to reach a position inside the right ventricle, see Figure 10-2. Another method that is occasionally used attaches the tips of the pacing wire to the outside surface of the right ventricle. A pacemaker with a single wire inserted into the right ventricle is called a ventricular pacemaker. A new brand of pacemaker with certain advantages for some patients utilizes two pacing wires. One is positioned in the right ventricle and the other in the right atrium and is called an atrioventricular pacemaker.

Prior to 1972, a power source for the pacemaker was derived from batteries that were chiefly mercury-zinc. These were heavy and lasted two to four years. The late 1970s showed

# Figure 10-2 Artificial Pacemaker

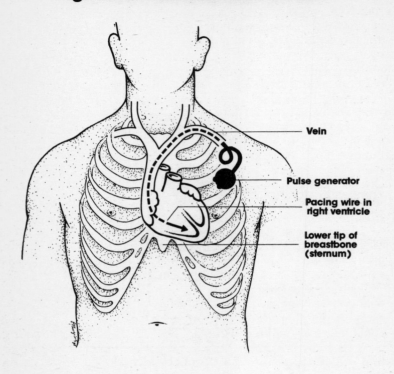

Vein

Pulse generator

Pacing wire in
right ventricle

Lower tip of
breastbone
(sternum)

major advances in electronics, and now virtually all pacemakers
are powered by varieties of lithium batteries. The life of the
lithium pacemakers varies from seven to ten years. Each patient is given a card that documents the type, model, serial
number, date of installation, and approximate life of the
pacemaker.

The patients are strongly advised to attend a pacemaker
clinic for follow-up in order to detect the rare occurrence of

pacemaker malfunction, and occasionally the pacemaker rate has to be adjusted. Most modern pacemakers are programmable. That is, by placing a device on the skin over the generator, radio signals are delivered to the pacer circuitry. This simple procedure is done in the cardiologist's office or a pacemaker clinic. The patients are usually followed for six to twelve weeks after the pacemaker is inserted, then twice annually. If signs of power-source depletion are observed, the patient is then seen monthly. Power-source depletion is easily detected as a decrease in rate when the system is monitored by passing a magnet over the generator. Batteries are changed every seven to ten years depending on the make of the pacemaker. The procedure requires very minor surgery. The flap of skin is lifted and the pacemaker generator is replaced. Pacemakers are programmed so that they work only when the patient's heart beats slowly, below the set rate. Pacemakers of the 1980s are electrically shielded so that it is no longer necessary to avoid electrical equipment as was the case with older pacemaker systems.

## Activities

Patients are allowed to exercise freely to the extent of their tolerance. Many are able to jog one to five miles daily and do similar exercises if angina or heart failure are not present. A patient with a pacemaker can lead a normal life.

# One Man's Story

OW, age forty-seven, was sitting watching television when he suddenly felt a pain in the center of his chest. The pain felt like nothing he had ever experienced before. The entire lower two-thirds of his breastbone and part of his left chest felt as if someone were crushing him in a vice. He started to feel weak and afraid, and he loosened his collar to relieve the feeling of strangulation. He called his wife for some antacid for what he assumed must be terrible indigestion due to the high-fat meal he had eaten thirty minutes earlier. Two antacid tablets did not relieve the pain and he started to pace restlessly around the room. He soon became dizzy, felt faint, and was forced to lie down. The pain was not relieved by lying flat, so his wife propped him up and started rubbing his back. About seven to ten minutes went by and the pain was becoming worse; he felt as if he was going to die. Though a sense of panic was beginning to set in, he did not want to alarm his wife. The passage of his entire life seemed to float before him. He was determined to sit up and to walk to see if it would ease the pain. He moved across the room, the dizziness was less than before, but the pain was of the same intensity. Both arms, from the shoulders to below the elbows, were now aching as if he carried a fifty-pound weight in each hand. There was no pain in his back. He tried to analyze what could be the reason for this pain. He had not done any physical work in the past month. It could easily be stomach upset since there was some discomfort at the lower end of his breastbone and stomach (epigastric area). He had been under pressure at work for the last month. His job was on the line and he was determined to show his colleagues and boss that he could cope. He had faced similar ˙stressful situations before. Suddenly, as he was wondering about the past, the pain became excruciating, constricting his chest. He could no longer hide his fear; his wife noticed his face had become pale. She dashed for the phone and called an ambulance, which came twenty minutes later. The wait was agonizing as his breathing and strangling sensation worsened. He had no nitroglycerin in the house since he was not known to have coronary heart disease. As soon as the ambulance arrived, an oxygen mask was applied and he was rushed to the emergency room of the nearest hospital. A diagnosis of an acute myocardial infarction was made and he was admitted to the coronary care unit of our hospital. He made a reasonable recovery and was discharged on the tenth hospital day. He did have mild heart failure during the first two days in the hospital but this cleared quickly. A few days after his attack, I placed him on a beta-blocker, propranolol, and a drug to try to prevent blood clotting, sulfinpyrazone. He discontinued his two-pack-a-day smoking habit. His cholesterol was 280 mg/dL, that is, mildly elevated. He was not overweight but he was placed on a diet with low cholesterol and low saturated fat; moderate salt restriction was appropriate. He was advised on an exercise program. He had liked jogging in the past, and three months after his heart attack, he was able to jog one to three miles daily. He did well for the next two years, during which time he took his medications regularly. He continued his exercise program doing three to ten miles daily, six days weekly. About eighteen months later, while standing in line at the bank he suddenly dropped to the floor. Fortunately, a trained nurse was in the line and cardiopulmonary resuscitation was commenced. He was resuscitated and rushed to the hospital. He was found to have complete heart block and a permanent pacemaker was inserted. He was discharged from the hospital a few days later and resumed his daily exercises.

About one year later, while on vacation, he suddenly experienced central chest pain that was similar to his first heart attack; he was rushed to the hospital. His attack was complicated by heart failure. His heart failure was cleared by the use of digoxin, a water pill, furosemide, and a vasodilator drug called captopril. Investigations showed that he had developed an aneurysm, a small swelling of part of the heart muscle.

He wanted to get back on an exercise program. Though at this stage he was not the best candidate for exercise, he started slowly over the next few weeks by walking one to three miles. He eased into jogging a quarter mile daily, but when he tried to do a half mile, he started getting shortness of breath and pain in the chest. This pain was immediately relieved by stopping the run. Angina was present and he now agreed to have a catheter study. Coronary arteriography was done, and this showed a complete block in one artery, more than 80 percent obstruction in two branches, and a small aneurysm of the left ventricle. He underwent coronary artery bypass surgery with three bypass grafts and repair of the aneurysm. Two weeks later, he was discharged from the hospital. He slowly began an exercise program, and ten months later he was once again jogging one to two miles daily. He completed the Terry Fox 10 Km Fun Run in September 1985.

## CORONARY ARTERY BYPASS SURGERY

Coronary artery bypass surgery is usually not done during the first few days after a heart attack except in rare instances. Usually, surgery is deferred for at least three months. However, in some centers, selective patients with a heart attack may have emergency coronary artery bypass grafts (CABG). Blood is brought in with a vein graft attached to the aorta and inserted below the point of the blockage in the artery, i.e., bypassing the blockage (Figure 11-1). Preliminary results of such surgery appear favorable; however, this procedure is presently experimental, and by 1990, the role of surgery during an acute heart attack may be better defined. Certainly, surgery can be done only in a select few since such sophisticated surgical facilities may never become widespread owing to the extraordinary cost and manpower necessary to maintain a surgical team and operating room around the clock. Aortocoronary bypass graft, discussed in Chapter 11, is indicated mainly to relieve the chest pain of angina pectoris.

## HUMAN HEART TRANSPLANTS

Since Christiaan Barnard performed the first human heart transplant in 1967, success has been achieved in a substantial number of instances, encouraging enough to persuade various centers to engage in a heart transplant program. However, despite recent breakthroughs to combat the rejection process, this problem has not been conquered. There is hope that by the 1990s the results of massive research on the rejection process and its suppression will provide solid answers and most importantly drugs that will suppress rejection without causing harm and suffering to patients. The next major drawback with any proposed heart transplant operation is the question of the donor's heart size. The transplant cannot be achieved if the donor's heart is too large for the recipient's heart cavity.

At present, heart transplants must be considered an experimental procedure; it is nevertheless essential for learning and may benefit mankind and help a select few.

Apart from fighting the rejection process, the availability of human donor hearts of appropriate size will always present problems, thus limiting heart transplants to a few individuals.

## ARTIFICIAL HEART

The artificial heart is on the horizon. It is a feasible approach and will be mastered given time. Consider that pacemakers, when developed in 1955, were 100 times the size of pacemakers produced in the late 1980s. They weighed about 250 grams whereas at present the size is that of a large coin and the weight about 40 grams. The size, weight, and electronics of the artificial heart will be improved to make the project feasible perhaps by the turn of the century. In the meantime, the project in a few U.S. centers remains experimental and should not be entertained as possible treatment except for the few who wish to participate in the experiments. The public must understand that the knowledge acquired from human experiments would assist centers in development of a small functional artificial heart. Such a device will need to be tested over several years to document its value and justify the cost. Such successes in medicine are usually followed by competing manufacturers providing original modifications and designs. In addition, cost, manpower, and feasibility limits the use of the artificial heart to very few patients and thus plays a limited role in the prevention of suffering and prolongation of life. An added role for a successful artificial heart is to support the patient until a suitable donor heart is available.

Several major problems must be rectified:

1. The psychological impact of an artificial heart transplant is a major obstacle. If no suitable donor is available, it becomes emotionally traumatic and stressful for the patient, family, and surgeons to risk removing the heart even when that heart is terminally diseased.
2. Experimenters must develop a machine that is small enough to fit into the chest cavity. This is not impossible.
3. The right ventricle pumps blood at a systolic blood pressure of 15 to 30 mm Hg whereas the left ventricle pumps at 100 to 140 mm Hg. The right and left side of artificial chambers will need to pump at different pressures and vary according to the activity of the individual—this is not impossible to achieve either, given time.

4. The materials used to coat the interior of the artificial heart should have the characteristics of the smooth endothelium lining of the normal heart. Blood particles and clots do not adhere to the smooth endothelial lining of the natural heart, whereas some artificial hearts in animals develop an aggregation of fibroblasts and endothelial cells (pannus) that obstruct the flow of blood through the right ventricle. In addition, complications may develop in animals that live for periods longer than ten months. Experiments are necessary in suitable animals other than calves, so as to extend testing beyond six months. Calves outgrow the pumping capacity of the transplant by the age of six months.

Various biological materials, including collagen, are being tested. However, even a collagen-lined heart if developed would not be continuously repaired and replaced. The normal heart and its lining is continuously repaired and replaced. Investigations are underway to develop methodology for producing a biological lining made up of living cells that can withstand the trauma caused by the blood's velocity and turbulence. An intriguing possibility is to find methods to cover the interior and exterior of the artificial heart with living cells derived from the recipient in the months prior to surgery. The key to such a feat lies in the yet unknown mechanisms controlling cell differentiation and growth. Such a miracle discovery may save the day and many lives. However, the area of organ reconstruction from natural elements may be as difficult to master as is the delineation of the exact cause of atherosclerosis and coronary thrombosis. Perhaps by the year 2100, instead of the artificial heart, the individual may sport a replaceable natural heart developed from his or her tissues. Ripley's believe it or not!

# CHAPTER 11

---

# ANGINA PECTORIS

## DEFINITIONS

Angina pectoris is not in itself a disease such as diabetes or pneumonia. It is the name used for the symptoms of chest pain of very short duration that originate from the heart muscle because of a relative lack of blood supply to the muscle.

The coronary arteries supply blood containing oxygen, glucose, and other nutrients to the heart muscle. Figure 1-1 shows the typical narrowing of a coronary artery by atherosclerosis. The internal diameter of the three main coronary arteries is only about the size of a soda straw. Even if the obstruction by a plaque of atheroma is severe, more than 75 percent narrowing, the heart muscle is still able to receive adequate amounts of oxygen when the heart is at rest and beating normally at about 70 beats per minute. However, during activities or under emotional stress, the heart rate may increase from 70 to reach 100 or more beats per minute; the blood pressure also increases, resulting in extra work for the heart muscle. To accomplish extra work, the heart muscle requires more oxygen. The obstruction in the artery causes insufficient blood with oxygen to reach the muscle to satisfy its needs during the vital few minutes. This temporary lack of blood to the heart muscle is called ischemia and herein is derived the medical name for the disease, ischemic heart disease, which is synonymous with coronary artery disease or coronary heart disease (CHD). Ischemia is defined as a local and temporary deficiency of blood.

Oxygen lack to the heart muscle is manifested by:

1. Chest pain called angina pectoris.
2. Changes on the electrocardiogram (ECG, EKG) that are recognized by the doctor as due to oxygen lack to the muscle. The ECG changes can occur without the patient feeling pain. (See Figure 6-2, "The Heart Under Stress.")

William Heberden in 1768 gave a detailed description of a peculiar type of chest discomfort suffered by his patients and he adopted the term "angina pectoris." His description was most appropriate. He wrote:

There is a disorder of the breasts marked with strong and peculiar symptoms, considerable for the kind of danger belonging to it, and not extremely rare which deserves to be mentioned more at length. The site of it, and the sense of strangling, and anxiety with which it is attended, may make it not improperly called angina pectoris.

They who are affected with it, are seized while they are walking (more especially if it be uphill, and soon after eating) with a painful and most disagreeable sensation in the breasts, which seems as if it were to extinguish life, if it were to increase or continue; but the moment they stand still all this uneasiness vanishes.

In all other respects, the patients are, at the beginning of this disorder, perfectly well, and in particular have no shortness of breath, from which it is totally different. The pain is sometimes situated in the upper part, sometimes in the middle, sometimes at the bottom of the os sterni, and often more inclined to the left than to the right. It likewise very frequently extends from the breasts to the middle of the left arm.

## Symptoms and Signs

The typical features of angina pectoris that enable the doctor to make the diagnosis are the following:

The relationship between the pain and the precipitating factor.

The pain always gets better within a few seconds or minutes when the precipitating activity is stopped. For example, the individual is quite well but on walking up an incline, especially against the wind, he or she develops discomfort in the chest. If the individual immediately stops the walk and rests a minute, thus allowing the heart work to decrease, the discomfort disappears immediately (within seconds to minutes). This concept of oxygen supply versus its demand by the heart muscle is the hallmark of angina. The doctor will ask about your symptoms and will try to draw this information from you. You can make a long list of what precipitates the pain and what relieves it, but the one important clue to help you and your doctor is that the pain or discomfort is precipitated by a particular activity, and once you stop the activity, the pain disappears within minutes.

## Activities that Precipitate Angina

1. A walk up a hill.
2. Walking against the wind.
3. Running with some associated anxiety for a bus or plane especially while carrying a bag. Anxiety is made more profound if the individual is late and must rush the run. Thus there is exertion and emotional stress.
4. A brisk walk or similar exertion soon after eating. This does not include bending and stooping, which can precipitate indigestion.
5. Unaccustomed exertion.
6. Emotional distress; for example, bad news, a scare, anger, rage, nightmares, and the like.
7. Overwhelming excitement; for example, watching your team playing football, hockey, baseball, basketball, and similar arousing programs can precipitate episodes of angina.

Note that I have not included activities such as walking upstairs, vacuuming, and housework, because these activities can produce pain from the chest wall, and if the individual can walk up a hill or one mile briskly, then walking up two flights of

stairs will not cause angina. Therefore, I never make a diagnosis
of angina based on a complaint of pain only on walking upstairs
or vacuuming.

## The Location of the Pain

The pain of angina is felt usually over or under the breastbone (retrosternal). Pain or discomfort extends over an area
usually the size of a fist and not an area as small as one or two
fingertips (see Chapter 10 for a detailed description of heart
attack pain). Occasionally pain may occur in the upper part of
the stomach just at the lower tip of the breastbone or the neck,
jaw, arms, elbows, or wrists, without pain being present in the
chest. Occasionally the elbow region escapes, and the individual feels the discomfort in the upper arm and a tingling feeling
in the fingers. The location of pain is not as important as the
cessation of pain on stopping the precipitating activity.

## Radiation of the Pain

Pain or discomfort may remain in an area about the size of
a fist felt under any part of the breastbone, but may move, that
is, radiate to be felt in the throat or jaw, arms, and hands.
Radiation is similar to that described for a heart attack (see
Figure 10-1). In some, pain may start in the arm and a few
seconds later be felt in the chest.

## Character of the Pain

The sensation may be perceived as pain but in many it is
only a discomfort or funny feeling that is difficult to describe.
The discomfort may be characterized as a tightness, pressure,
heaviness, constriction, strangulation, or choking in the throat.
Occasionally it is a burning, an ache in the jaw, shortness of
breath, or a feeling of nausea. The discomfort can produce a
strangling, frightened feeling that often bothers the individual
more than discomfort.

## Duration of the Pain

The pain or discomfort of angina usually lasts one to three minutes and occasionally about five minutes. The duration is rarely less than thirty seconds. Importantly the pain rarely lasts fifteen to twenty minutes; this may occur in individuals in whom the obstruction in the coronary artery has progressed. Pain lasting more than twenty minutes should not be called angina because it is no longer a temporary lack of blood supply. Pain more than twenty minutes should be assessed in the emergency room because it can be due to a heart attack or causes other than the heart.

## Relief of the Pain

Stopping the precipitating activity is nearly always successful. Also, angina is usually, but not always, relieved within one to two minutes by a tablet of nitroglycerin under the tongue (sublingual). However, other causes of chest pain may last less than two minutes and pain other than that due to angina, esophageal spasm for example, may be relieved by nitroglycerin. Other causes of chest pain that may be confused with angina or heart pain are discussed in Chapter 10.

To reemphasize, angina is caused by a temporary lack of blood supply to the heart muscle. A temporary lack of blood supply to a segment of heart muscle is usually due to a temporarily increased demand for oxygen that cannot be achieved because of significant obstruction (more than 75 percent) of a coronary artery by atherosclerosis. The hardened artery cannot expand or dilate and not enough blood passes the obstruction to meet the demand. In addition, spasm or constriction of a small segment of a coronary artery is a well-known cause of angina. The spasm can occur in a completely normal artery or at the site of a partially obstructing plaque of atheroma. Coronary artery spasm and the cause of angina will be discussed shortly. The good news is that during the few seconds of oxygen deprivation, the small segment of heart muscle is not damaged; there is no death of cells. The muscle is under strain, but once sufficient blood supply is reestablished to meet the needs of the muscle, the strain and pain disappear. It is reassuring news that the muscle remains functionally and structurally normal. An individual may have 100 episodes of angina per year and yet no damage to the muscle occurs. Damage only occurs when the artery is completely blocked by atherosclerosis and clots, causing a heart attack (myocardial infarction) (see Figure 1-1).

## Classifications

Angina is usually classified as:

Stable angina.
Unstable angina.
Angina due to coronary artery spasm.

You must understand a few basic definitions of angina to appreciate the management schedules.

### Stable Angina

Angina is described as stable when there has been no change in the past sixty days in the frequency of attacks, duration (less than ten minutes), or precipitating causes. There is no pain at rest except if caused by emotional distress. I must emphasize that for angina to occur at least one coronary artery must have a narrowing of greater than 75 percent.

### Unstable Angina

Angina is described as unstable when there is a change in pattern, an increase in frequency, severity and/or duration of pain, and a lesser degree of known precipitating factors. For example, JM, age fifty-three, was late for a dental appointment, and he had to search for a space to park his car. He had tried two parking lots then finally had to squeeze in closely between two cars. He felt a bit sweaty and had a funny sensation in the upper part of his chest for a few seconds but brushed this aside.

He was about 400 yards away from the dentist office; it was a rather cold November day and the wind was fierce. He dashed across the street and was suddenly stopped by a strange pressure in his chest as if it were being squeezed tight. He kept on walking but half a minute later, the discomfort was a moderate pain. He hurried into the building and had to lean against the wall and take deep breaths. He opened his neck button and tie and felt better in about half a minute. He had a root canal done without any problems and went home feeling fairly well. He remained quite well until a few weeks later, while walking briskly up a hill, he experienced pain that was relieved only when he stopped his walk. He went to his doctor, who made the diagnosis of angina pectoris and he was given nitroglycerin tablets to take sublingually if pain recurred. The pain occurred only twice during the next year and only on moderate exertion such as brisk two-mile walks or a half-mile walk on a cold, windy day, or occasionally while walking uphill. There was never pain at rest. However, two years later he noticed that his pain would last four to five minutes instead of the usual half to one minute. He started having pain on walking short distances, i.e., 200 yards, even on a good day. Mild pain occurred a few times on intercourse and at times while looking at a hockey game. He visited his doctor, who gave him oral nitrate tablets to take four times daily. However, within two weeks he started having pain on walking twenty to fifty yards and pain would come on even with rest. The pain at rest lasted ten to twenty minutes, which frightened him and he went to our emergency room. A diagnosis was made: Stable angina for three or more years, but unstable angina for about two weeks. He was admitted to our hospital because of unstable angina. Unstable angina can lead to a heart attack within a few weeks, whereas stable angina does so only occasionally and, in some patients, only after five to ten years. Therefore, beware of the changes in the pain pattern and changes in the duration or frequency of pain, especially, if the same kind of pain occurs at rest; even if it lasts less than twenty minutes, go to the emergency room.

## Coronary Artery Spasm

Transient constriction, or spasm of a coronary artery, is a definite cause of angina; however, it is fortunately rare. It may occur in patients older than age thirty-five and comes on mainly at rest. Therefore, some physicians use the term "variant angina." The individual may never have pain on minimal or vigorous exertion. Thus, the condition is entirely different from the common type of angina caused by atherosclerosis obstructing a coronary artery. Pain usually lasts one to fifteen minutes and is usually relieved by one to three nitroglycerin tablets. Coronary artery spasm can occur at any time of the day but is most common at night and in the early hours of the morning. The patient may awaken with pain. Rarely, exertion, alcohol, or aspirins can precipitate attacks. Recently a new group of drugs, calcium antagonists, have been developed and have been shown to be very successful in treating this condition. Occasionally, a patient with obstruction of the coronary arteries by atheroma gets spasm at the site of a plaque and may therefore have pain on exertion and at rest. Such patients are therefore treated as unstable angina.

# WHAT INVESTIGATIONS ARE NECESSARY?

1. Resting electrocardiogram.
2. A stress test.
3. Chest X-ray.
4. Coronary arteriography (arteriogram).
5. Nuclear scans.
6. Echocardiogram.
7. Holter monitor.

These procedures are discussed below.

Angina produces no abnormal physical signs or findings that the doctor can detect with his or her usual examination. Therefore, the patient's story or history is of great importance in making the diagnosis.

1. **The electrocardiogram** at rest in patients with angina is often normal but can show signs of chronic oxygen lack (ischemia) or an old scar of a healed myocardial infarct. The ECG may show disturbances of the heart rhythm, i.e., extra beats and electrical disturbances as well as heart enlargement. To reemphasize, the ECG is a valuable test for patients with or without heart disease, but a normal ECG does not mean that the individual does not have angina. Therefore, to capture the changes on the ECG, it must be done during the pain (a rare occurrence) or during an exercise stress test. The resting ECG may show the following abnormalities:

a. An old heart attack, which has caused a residual scar in the heart muscle.

b. Chronic ischemic changes due to oxygen lack or changes that indicate that the left ventricle is working under strain.

c. Electrical disturbances such as blocks in the electrical bundles called right or left bundle branch block or heart block.

d. Extra beats, i.e., ventricular premature beats.

e. Enlargement of the left ventricle or the left atrium.

f. A very weak area or bulge of the heart muscle (aneurysm).

   The ECG may show a very slow heart rate, which may indicate disease of the sinus node generator (pacemaker). If a prior ECG is available, a comparison in pattern is most useful. Therefore, it is wise for heart patients who are traveling outside the country or state to carry an electrocardiogram during their travels. This may prevent holdup in emergency rooms and hasten discharge from hospital.

2. **A stress test** usually helps to confirm the diagnosis and can be used for future reference to detect the progression of the coronary artery disease. Other aspects of the stress test are discussed in Chapter 5, "Exercise."

3. **A chest X-ray** is usually normal in patients with angina.

4.   **Indications for coronary arteriography** (arteriograms or angiograms) include the following:

a.   The most important reason to have this test is the presence of angina that interferes with lifestyle to such an extent that it is deemed unacceptable by the patient and the physician. The majority of patients with stable angina are able to live with the occasional occurrence of the fleeting chest discomfort that they know will be precipitated by a particular exertion or emotion. They realize that the pain does not damage the heart muscle and that on stopping the precipitating activity, pain or discomfort disappears immediately or is quickly relieved by a nitroglycerin tablet. Such patients may learn to live with angina from one to twenty years, and nothing else is done. Symptoms can be further improved in many by the use of beta-blockers and in some with the addition of calcium antagonists. The combination of drugs greatly reduces the occurrence of chest pain. In a few patients with stable angina, pain may occur daily and can interfere with work or lifestyle. Despite the fleeting nature of the pain, the patient may not be satisfied to live with this annoyance and may ask, "What else can be done?" The doctor in many cases may suggest that a coronary arteriogram be done. Thus the doctor-patient relationship is of utmost importance in patients with angina.

b.   Patients with unstable angina will need arteriography within a few weeks or months after their pain has subsided. The majority of these patients will need to undergo coronary artery bypass surgery. However, if surgery is contraindicated because of other medical problems or age, then there is little point to submit the patient to the test.

c.   In patients with heart attacks, it is important to have the arteriography done within the first two or three hours, so that drugs can be quickly given into the blocked coronary artery. However, as mentioned earlier, newer drugs are becoming available that appear to be effective when given simply through a vein in the arm. Therefore, coronary arteriography may not be necessary when proof becomes available that this method is effective. Hopefully, the appropriate method of giving these drugs will be clarified by 1987.

d.  There are a few patients in whom the diagnosis of angina is confusing, especially when symptoms or reflux esophagitis make the diagnosis difficult. Coronary arteriograms may be necessary to unravel the mystery and prevent patients from becoming cardiac cripples.

To reemphasize, the main reason for having a coronary arteriogram is to show what part of the coronary artery is blocked and to what extent so as to determine whether the individual is a candidate for coronary artery bypass surgery. Therefore, I always ensure that the patient is, first, a suitable candidate for surgery, that is, that the angina is severe enough that he or she will need to undergo surgery to relieve the pain, and, second, that there are no medical conditions such as severe bronchitis that may contraindicate surgery. As well, patients over seventy-five are rarely submitted to cardiac surgery.

Coronary arteriography remains the most important method of defining the presence and severity of atherosclerosis of the coronary artery. This test also reveals the size and shape of the left ventricle as well as its ability to contract evenly and forcibly, the presence and size of a bulge in the left ventricle (aneurysm), and problems with valves in the heart. More than 500,000 coronary arteriograms are performed in the United States annually. The procedure is not painful, and depending on the center, the patient is usually admitted the night before, the tests are done the next day, and the patient is discharged later that afternoon. In some institutions, facilities exist for a substantial number of patients to have the test done during the day with discharge several hours later if the condition is satisfactory. The patient is usually advised not to eat solid food after midnight on the day of the examination. Fluids are allowed up to one hour prior to the procedure. The patient is sedated with 5 mg of diazepam (Valium) given orally, and a specially made catheter is introduced either into the right arm artery (brachial artery) under local anesthesia or the artery in the groin (femoral artery). A small opening is made in the artery and a pigtail-like catheter is introduced and passed under X-ray guidance to the aorta and finally to the area where the aorta leaves the heart. At this point, the coronary arteries usually branch from the aorta, and the catheter is directed into the left and then the right coronary artery. A dye is injected and can be visualized by means of several X-rays taken in different planes. The X-rays will show the heart and arteries, the normal arteries or ones with blockage by plaques of atheroma similar to those depicted in Figure 1-1. Most importantly, any blockage in the coronary artery is clearly visualized. Coronary arteriography is a relatively safe procedure in experienced hands when done in well-equipped laboratories. Mortality is less than 0.1 percent and minor complications are rare. However, because the procedure is not without complications, the test must be justifiable and the patient must be aware of the risks attached. Patients are usually very keen to have the procedure since they understand it is the only way to know, without doubt, the extent and severity of the coronary obstruction. As well, surgery cannot be done without first visualizing the vessels (an X-ray movie is made and can be replayed during surgery to show the blockages).

5. **Nuclear scans** include (a) the thallium scan, and (b) the gated cardiac scan (cardiac blood pool).

a. The thallium scan is useful in selected patients with angina to show the areas of the heart muscle that are poorly perfused with blood. The technique is simple, nonpainful, and reliable. During an exercise stress test, usually on the treadmill, a known minute amount of radio isotope, thallium-201, is injected into a vein. The thallium reaches the heart and is distributed through the coronary arteries. The areas of the heart muscle that are not receiving adequate blood flow because of blockage of the coronary arteries will receive less thallium, and these areas can be seen on a video screen. The thallium test is usually indicated when the exercise stress test is not conclusive or is abnormal in an individual who has no symptoms, or in patients with left bundle branch block, since in this condition, the electrocardiogram and stress test cannot evaluate the areas of oxygen lack. Thus, nuclear scans represent an important relatively noninvasive testing method that provide very useful information.

b.     Another relatively noninvasive test that gives a good estimation of how much blood the heart ejects with each beat is the gated cardiac scan. With each beat, the normal heart expels at least 50 percent of the blood contained in each ventricle. The percentage ejected is called the ejection fraction, and it is one of the best indicators of the efficiency and strength of heart contraction. The normal ejection fraction is between 50 and 75 percent. The ejection fraction is one of the most important measures used by the cardiologist to judge the strength or functional capacity of the heart. The ejection fraction is accurately measured during coronary arteriography, and with a similar degree of accuracy, it can be determined with the gated cardiac pool study. In this test a radioisotope, technetium, is injected into an arm vein; the isotope binds to red blood cells and reaches the chambers of the heart. In particular, the left ventricle is well seen with sophisticated scintillation cameras and the data is processed by computer. The force of contraction and the motion of the heart muscle wall is visualized on a video screen. If the muscle is contracting poorly or contracting abnormally, as might be expected with an aneurysm, this can be detected in many cases.

6.     An echocardiogram is a painless, noninvasive diagnostic technique that utilizes ultrasound. It gives the cardiologist a superb, simple, no-risk evaluation of the valves of the heart, the heart muscle, the types of force and contraction, and the determination of the ejection fraction. The size of each chamber can be measured, and in particular, enlargement of the heart muscle and the position of the septum can be easily defined.

Most individuals have heard of the use of ultrasound for the detection of submarines (naval sonar) as well the whales' and dolphins' reliance on ultrasound, not vision. The application of ultrasound in the area of obstetrics to detect the normal and abnormal fetus and problems in the pelvis during pregnancy is well known.

The echocardiogram does not assist in the diagnosis of stable or unstable angina, and normal or blocked coronary arteries cannot be visualized by ultrasound. However, because the muscle contraction can be visualized, echocardiography is used in some patients with an acute heart attack to detect special complications.

7. **The Holter monitor** is occasionally utilized in patients with angina. The machine, about the size of a pocket, records a continuous twenty-four- to forty-eight-hour electrocardiogram. The instrument is strapped to the waist, and the patient returns home and carries on all normal activities, as well as sleep. After twenty-four or forty-eight hours, the machine is returned to the doctor's office. The tape is played and a recording is made. The doctor studies the tracings and determines the number of extra beats (extrasystoles) that occurred during this period and whether or not the extra beats require treatment. The test is requested when patients with angina complain of palpitations, or when the doctor detects extra beats on listening with the stethoscope or sees such disturbances of rhythm on the electrocardiogram or during stress testing.

## WHICH DRUGS ARE USEFUL TO TREAT ANGINA?

1. Nitrates, nitroglycerin: sublingual, buccal against the gum, and preparations applied to the skin. Nitrates taken orally.
2. Beta-blockers.
3. Calcium antagonists.

*Nitrates*

## Nitroglycerin; Glyceryl Trinitrate

Supplied: Sublingual nitroglycerin tablets: 0.15, 0.3, and 0.6 mg. Sublingual glyceryl trinitrate tablets: 300, 500, and 600 micrograms (mcg).

Dosage: The patient is advised to start with 0.15 mg or 0.3 mg as a test dose. The tablet is placed under the tongue with the patient seated. The drug will not be as effective if the patient is lying down, and if the patient is standing, dizziness or faintness may occur. Thereafter, the usual prescribed dose is 0.6 mg of nitroglycerin or 500 to 600 mcg glyceryl trinitrate. The 0.6 mg is advisable except:

1. If the systolic blood pressure on routine follow-up is 110 mm Hg or less and it is felt that the larger dose may decrease the blood pressure too low to less than 100 mm Hg.
2. If there is patient sensitivity causing severe headaches. Headaches are due to dilatation of the arteries in the scalp and not to an increase in blood pressure.

Patients are instructed that nitroglycerin tablets are to be kept in a dark place in light-protected bottles; they may be rendered useless after three to six months if they are not protected from light. Patients are advised to have at least two bottles available. These two bottles must contain approximately one month's supply, and the absorbent cotton should be removed to ensure rapid availability in emergencies. At the end of each month, the tablets should be discarded and the supply replenished from a third stock bottle. The stock bottle should be well stoppered and kept in a cool place at a temperature between 40 and 80°F (10 and 25°C). In areas where the temperature exceeds 86°F (30°C), the stock bottle should be kept in the refrigerator but not the freezer. Tablets should not be kept in pill boxes. Occasionally, check the activity of the tablets; if they are good, they cause a burning, stinging feeling under the tongue and a headache.

Patients are advised to take one tablet before activities known to precipitate pain. If pain is not relieved by one tablet, a second tablet is taken five minutes after the first. If there is no relief, the patient should immediately go to an emergency department. I must reemphasize that nitroglycerin relieves the pain of angina but not the pain of a heart attack.

## HOW DOES NITROGLYCERIN WORK?

The drug dilates veins, especially in the lower half of the body; therefore, blood pools in veins of the lower limbs and abdomen, and less blood reaches the heart. The heart's work and oxygen requirements are temporarily reduced, and thus, pain is relieved. If the individual is lying flat, only minimal amounts of blood can pool in the legs, and nitroglycerin is less effective. Nitroglycerin also works by causing mild dilatation of the coronary arteries and so relieves pain. When arteries are hardened by atherosclerosis, dilatation of rigid arteries is only occasionally possible. The drug causes a mild decrease in blood pressure because it causes slight dilation of arteries, and a mild increase in heart rate may occur, causing the heart to pound a little harder.

## MUST YOU USE NITROGLYCERIN, AND HOW MANY TABLETS ARE TOO MUCH?

It is not necessary to use the nitroglycerin tablets if your pain subsides in a few seconds after discontinuation of the precipitating activity. Nitroglycerin takes about one to two minutes to become effective and lasts about fifteen minutes. Many patients get to know that slowing or stopping certain activities eases discomfort and therefore they do not take nitroglycerin. However, even these patients should keep nitroglycerin handy. If pain is known to last more than two minutes, then the individual should take a nitroglycerin as soon as the discomfort begins. Nitroglycerin is safe, and the more quickly it is taken the better. In patients in whom one tablet does not completely relieve the pain, a second is taken five minutes after the first tablet. It is rare to need more than two tablets to get complete relief if the pain is due to angina.

Individuals who have recurrent pain lasting one to ten minutes once or twice a week will usually need to take four to six nitroglycerin weekly, and a few patients take more than fourteen tablets a week. If you are taking more than ten tablets a week, you should speak to your doctor because it is possible that other medications could be added to prevent the pain. A referral to a cardiologist is advisable. Also, patients who need to take more than sixty tablets per month may well be taking tablets for pain that is not coming from the heart. The majority of patients with angina take one to thirty nitroglycerins per month. I certainly do not allow my patients to take more than thirty nitroglycerins per month since I would then consider treatment to be inadequate. I would recommend the addition of beta-blockers, and after one to two months if there is no relief, calcium antagonists are added. If sufficient relief is not obtained, cardiac surgery is considered.

## Buccal Nitroglycerin

A new addition to nitrate therapy is a long-acting tablet that contains glyceryl trinitrate impregnated into an inert polymer matrix that allows slow, continuous release over four to five hours. The drug takes effect in one to five minutes and lasts from four to six hours. The tablets are placed *between the upper lip and gum* and dissolve within a few hours. They must *not* be chewed or swallowed. The advantage of this preparation over tablets of oral nitrates is that the active drug reaches the blood quickly by bypassing the liver and therefore attains better blood levels than tablets that are swallowed. However, because the tablets have to be kept between the upper lip and gum for a few hours, some patients do not like the inconvenience. The drug therefore is useful, but has a limited role. The trade names of these preparations are given in Appendix A.

Dosage: For treatment of angina: 1–2 mg two or three times daily before a precipitating activity. In severe angina, the dose of 3–5 mg is used.

For treatment of heart failure: 5 mg three times daily and at bedtime for the relief of shortness of breath.

These oral preparations held in the mouth (buccal) play a small role and compete with the use of other nitroglycerin preparations applied to the skin.

## Cutaneous Nitroglycerins

A paste or ointment and, recently, long-acting or slow-release cutaneous nitroglycerin applied to the skin have become available. The paste and ointment, which must not be massaged into the skin, are messy and have variable effects. On the other hand, slow-release cutaneous preparations made in the form of Band-Aids or the like, are clean and dry and can be used once daily. However, trials have not yet proven their reliability, and their cost must be justified.

The paste or ointment starts to work in thirty to sixty minutes and lasts from four to a maximum of six hours and from about eighteen to twenty-four hours with the long-acting Band-Aid or disklike preparations.

The cutaneous preparations should not be applied to the forearms, hands, or lower legs since it takes longer for the drug to reach the general circulation. These skin preparations are useful during dental work and for minor or major surgery in patients with coronary heart disease.

An attempt must be made by the doctor and patient to restrict the use of skin preparations to two to fourteen days (maximum of twenty-eight days). These drugs are not meant to be used for more than a few weeks since they lose their activity. In addition, these preparations must not be stopped suddenly—for example, after using them for a few days, the dose should be tapered and reduced slowly over the next one to two days. In a few patients when the drugs are stopped suddenly, angina or heart failure can become worse.

The various preparations are listed in Appendix A.

## Isosorbide Dinitrate

Supplied:
Sublingual tablets to be dissolved under the tongue: 2.5 mg, 5 mg, 10 mg.

Chewable tablets: 10 mg.
Tablets for oral use: 5 mg, 10 mg, 20 mg, 30 mg.
Prolonged-action tablets: 40 mg.
Prolonged-action capsules: 40 mg..

Dosage: A sublingual 5 mg tablet is dissolved under the tongue before an activity that is known to produce chest discomfort. The 10 mg tablet is taken four times daily on an empty stomach, e.g., one hour before meals. If headaches are not too severe, the drug can be increased to 15 mg four times daily for a few days or weeks, then 30 mg four times daily. The prolonged-action 40 mg preparation is taken once daily.

Advice and adverse effects: The sublingual 5 mg tablets take three to five minutes to become effective, somewhat longer than nitroglycerin; therefore, patients are advised to use nitroglycerin during an attack of angina. (Also, the drug is more expensive than nitroglycerin.) The drug's effect lasts from ten to thirty minutes. It is, therefore, not a long-acting preparation but it can be taken just the same as a nitroglycerin tablet prior to activity. For example, I may give a patient 5 mg sublingual isosorbide dinitrate at the tenth golf hole if he usually has chest discomfort on the eleventh hole.

The 10 mg tablet is relatively not effective. The 30 mg tablet has to be used at least four times daily, and often three hourly, to be of any value.[8] At this or higher doses, headaches and dizziness are common and many patients cannot tolerate doses of 40 and 60 mg four times daily, which is the type of dose needed to get relief. Importantly, the U.S. Food and Drug Administration (FDA) has classified all oral nitrates as only possibly effective and I concur with their report. The drug should not be used as first choice in the treatment of angina pectoris, especially since two preparations, beta-blockers and calcium antagonists, have proven to be effective and reliable. In addition, beta-blockers can prevent death or favorably alter the outcome of a heart attack. The use of oral nitrates, therefore, makes sense in patients who cannot take or do not respond to beta-blockers and/or calcium antagonists.

The addition of isosorbide dinitrate to beta-blockers and calcium antagonists can be regarded as polypharmacy; think of the patient, the cost, and the side effects of all three medications.[9]

## Isosorbide Mononitrate

The 5-mononitrate of isosorbide dinitrate has become available in Europe and achieves more consistent plasma nitrate levels. The drug may become available in the United States. Dosage: 20 mg two to three times daily after meals. Maintenance 20 to 40 mg twice daily.

## Other Oral Long-Acting Nitrates

Several drugs on the market in this category have been used since 1961. They contain varying quantities of glyceryl trinitrate or its derivatives. Such drugs include pentaerythritol tetranitrate and erythrityl tetranitrate. These are not recommended in view of their inconsistent antianginal effect. I discontinued the use of these preparations in 1966.

Additional side effects of oral nitrates include flushing of the skin, palpitations, incontinence, weakness, muscle twitching, perspiration, fainting, skin rash, and loss of hair. On occasion, prolonged use at high doses has been known to cause a defect in the hemoglobin of the blood.

## Caution and Drug Interaction of Nitrate Preparations

When combined with drugs that dilate arteries, such as prazosin and calcium antagonists such as nifedipine, rapid heartbeat, severe dizziness, and fainting may occur because of a marked fall in blood pressure. As well, use of alcohol may cause an excessive lowering of blood pressure. Prolonged use of nitrate preparations at high dosage may increase intraocular pressure and worsen glaucoma. Measurement of internal eye pressure is advisable for individuals with glaucoma who are taking high doses of nitrates for prolonged periods. If someone has glaucoma that is not under control, these drugs should be avoided.

## Beta-Blockers

Apart from nitroglycerin under the tongue, beta-blockers are the most beneficial drugs used in the treatment of angina. They have been in use in the United Kingdom since 1964 and in the United States since 1969. The first and most well-known drug in this group is propranolol (Inderal). Several beta-blockers have been approved by the FDA over the years, but they have few advantages over propranolol. The subtle differences will be discussed.

Beta-blockers block the effects of the stimulant stress hormones adrenaline and noradrenaline at the so-called beta-receptor sites present on the surface of cells in the heart and in some blood vessels. They therefore prevent the increase in heart rate, the force of heart muscle contraction, and the rise in blood pressure normally produced by these stimulants. Beta-blockers approved by the FDA are atenolol, nadolol, metoprolol, propranolol, pindolol, and timolol. Their role in the prevention of heart attack and death is discussed in Chapters 5 and 10. This discussion will center on their role in angina.

In patients with angina, at least one coronary artery has a block greater than 75 percent. At rest, sufficient blood reaches the heart muscle. However, during moderate activities, the heart rate and blood pressure increases and the heart muscle contracts more forcefully to do the work, because more blood containing oxygen is required. The blockage prevents an adequate supply of oxygen from reaching the muscle. This oxygen lack causes the heart muscle to become painful and the heart rate and blood pressure may further increase during the stress of pain. Basically beta-blockers cause the heart muscle to require less oxygen to do the same amount of work. The heart rate multiplied by the systolic blood pressure gives an estimation of the amount of work and oxygen required by the heart muscle. Beta-blockers decrease both heart rate and blood pressure, and therefore less oxygen is required. As well, they cause the heart muscle to contract less forcefully so that less oxygen is used. Importantly, these drugs divert blood from the areas of the heart that have an abundant supply to the deprived area. No other group of drugs possesses the remarkable properties that can produce such beneficial effects in patients with angina.

Nitrates increase heart rate and can shunt blood away from the deprived area. Beta-blockers should be the first oral drugs employed in the treatment of angina. It is surprising to this author that many patients take oral nitrates without beta-blockers and tolerate the headaches for little gain. In addition, I must reemphasize that oral nitrates do not prevent heart attacks or heart deaths. Most importantly, as outlined in Chapters 9 and 13, beta-blockers can prevent ventricular fibrillation and death; also, they reduce the recurrence rate of a second heart attack and can reduce the size of the heart attack.[9] I need not give you or your doctor further clues as to why beta-blockers are superior to oral nitrates. It is of interest that I had oral nitrates banned from our hospital in 1974. However, it is my distinct impression that older doctors still prescribe oral nitrates liberally before resorting to beta-blockers; the younger, recently graduated doctor resorts to the new wonder drugs, calcium antagonists, often before trying a beta-blocker. The merits of calcium antagonists will be discussed shortly.

## Use of Beta-Blockers

If there are *no* contraindications to the use of beta-blockers, the treatment of angina should be nitroglycerin sublingual plus a beta-blocker preferably given once and, at most, twice daily. The beta-blocker is always started at a very low dose and, over a period of days or weeks, increased to reach an effective dose. A low dose of propranolol, for example, 20 mg three times daily before meals increasing after a week or two to 40 mg three times daily, is advisable. The doctor will check to be sure that the pulse and blood pressure are stable and that there are no side effects from the medications. If necessary, the dose can be increased to 160 mg long-acting (LA) capsule once daily, or 160 mg in the morning and 80 mg at bedtime. A dose of less than 120 mg of propranolol is seldom of value, since only in a few would a dose of 80 mg block the effects of adrenaline and noradrenaline produced during emotional or physical stress. A few patients, 1 in 100, are very sensitive to beta-blockers and their pulse rate decreases to less than forty-eight per minute. It is extremely rare to learn of patients who come to harm because of a slow heart rate. However, a heart rate less than forty-two per minute may cause dizziness and the individual may be forced to lie down. The body quickly compensates and the effects of a 40 mg tablet wears off in about four hours. The doctor usually reduces the dose, or in very few cases, the drug is discontinued. The reader must understand that in North America there are more than 10 million individuals who are taking beta-blockers or who are candidates for such therapy. Thus, some of the discussions given in Chapters 9 and 13 are repeated here in a different format.

## General Cautions That Relate to All Beta-Blockers

1. *Do not suddenly stop taking beta-blockers.* If you have been taking a beta-blocker for several months, your heart rate and oxygen requirement is controlled in just the same way as the reins that control a horse. If beta-blockers are stopped abruptly, it is similar to cutting the reins; the horse may gallop away. Therefore, the heart rate may increase from the accustomed fifty-five to sixty-five per minute to eighty to ninety per minute; as well, the blood pressure may increase and impose sudden strain on the heart—this can precipitate angina. It is relatively safe to miss one dose of a beta-blocker, or at the most two doses per week. I certainly do not advise you to miss any doses, but there are always unavoidable circumstances. No harm usually results from one missed dose. However, omitting the drug for two to three days consecutively may precipitate angina. Withdrawals should be gradual over weeks and under the guidance of your doctor. Further discussion on withdrawal of beta-blockers is discussed in Chapter 13, "Hypertension."

2. If you are short of breath or wheezing, report this to your doctor as soon as possible.

3. Beta-blockers must not be used in combination with monoamine oxidase (MAO) inhibitors. Presently these drugs are only rarely used to treat some types of severe depression and this is generally not a problem in practice.

4. Do not take decongestants, or cold or cough remedies containing epinephrine (adrenaline), phenylephrine, or propranolamine. An increase in blood pressure can occur.

5. The combination of beta-blockers and digitalis (digoxin) is relatively safe but in a few individuals further slowing of the heart rate can occur. Therefore, the doses must be controlled carefully by your doctor. However, you should have no fear, because in clinical practice only 1 in 100 patients may have serious slowing of the heart rate.

6. The combination of a beta-blocker and a calcium antagonist, verapamil, can cause heart failure if the heart muscle is already weak.

7. Metoprolol and propranolol are broken down in the liver more rapidly in smokers so that blood levels of the drugs are reduced; thus, the drugs may be rendered useless. Atenolol and nadolol are not broken down in the liver and are not affected by smoking. Timolol has been shown to prevent heart attacks or death in smokers as well as nonsmokers.

8. Alcohol: two pints of beer or three ounces of liquor do not cause any interaction or alteration in effectiveness.

## Contraindications

*Do not take beta-blockers if you have any of the following:*

1. Heart failure: Your doctor will obviously know your problem and will not prescribe the drug if you have heart failure and require treatment for angina. However, the good news is that only few patients with angina have heart failure. Beta-blockers can precipitate heart failure in patients with very weak heart muscle function. However, I must point out that the heart muscle is the strongest muscle in the body. It does more work than any other muscle during an individual's lifetime. Many patients who have had two heart attacks are still able to engage in a brisk two-mile walk or climb three flights of stairs, and some can jog

one to three miles. The remaining heart muscle is stronger than the quadriceps muscle of the thigh. I refer you to Chapters 9 and 10, where I have discussed heart failure and beta-blockers in patients who have had a heart attack, and to Chapter 15, where the strength of the heart muscle is reemphasized. The heart muscle is strong enough in about 90 out of 100 patients with angina to allow the use of beta-blockers.

2. A very large heart, which signifies a very weak heart muscle. Fortunately patients with angina rarely have a very large heart.

3. Heart block or severe electrical disturbances of the heart (sick sinus syndrome), which causes very slow heartbeats. This occurs in about 1 in every 1,000 patients with angina, and beta-blockers are contraindicated.

4. In bronchial asthma, severe chronic bronchitis, or emphysema. In some patients who have mild chronic bronchitis and for whom beta-blockers are deemed necessary to control angina, the doctor usually chooses atenolol or metoprolol, which has less effect on the lungs. These two drugs are relatively safe at low doses.

5. Do not commence beta-blockers during a flare-up of allergic rhinitis.

6. Severe reduction of the arterial circulation to the legs and feet.

## Side Effects

1. The heart and vessels:
a. Precipitation of heart failure in patients with a very weak heart muscle, as discussed.
b. Severe slowing of the heart rate to less than forty-two beats per minute in rare cases if the drug dose is not carefully adjusted. This is usually quickly spotted by the symptoms of dizziness and ill feeling, and can be quickly rectified. Hence, in practice this is not a problem.
c. Cold hands and feet can occur in about 10 percent of patients. The condition improves immediately on discontinuation of the beta-blocker.

2. The lungs: Precipitation of wheezing and difficult breathing in individuals who are known to have allergic asthma or severe bronchitis.

3. The nervous or muscular system:

a. Dizziness due to excess slowing of the pulse and excessive reduction in blood pressure.

b. Vivid dreams, occurring in about 10 percent of patients taking propranolol. These usually clear when given an alternative medication such as atenolol, timolol, or nadolol.

c. Mild depression. Occurring in less than 10 percent of patients, it is not a major problem in practice. Since atenolol and nadolol do not get into the brain as does propranolol, they cause fewer problems.

d. Weakness and muscle fatigue of a varying degree, occurring in about 10 percent of patients. A change from propranolol to atenolol or nadolol is advisable. If symptoms persist and no other cause can be found, the beta-blockers should be discontinued. In my own large cardiology practice, I have found fewer than ten such patients since 1965. Certainly beta-blockers may affect individuals who wish to jog more than two miles, but then, patients with angina do not jog.

e. Reduction of libido and impotence. Although it occurs in less than 5 percent of patients, it must be monitored by patient and physician. However, beta-blockers, by decreasing the heart rate, blood pressure, and heart work can be useful if pain is precipitated by intercourse.

f. Stomach upset from beta-blockers, in less than 1 percent.

g. Other side effects: In some patients, insomnia, altered sleep patterns, nervousness, muscle cramps, and muscle joint pains can be caused by pindolol.[10]

## Antenolol

Supplied: Tablets: 50 mg, 100 mg.
Dosage: Start with ½ of a 50 mg tablet daily for about three days then 50 mg daily at any time of the day. If the condition warrants, the doctor often starts with 50 mg daily. Food does not interfere with the effectiveness of atenolol. One hundred

mg may be necessary if angina is not controlled and especially if the blood pressure is elevated.

Caution: In patients with kidney failure the dose should be reduced, e.g., to 50 mg every other day.

## Metoprolol

Supplied: Tablets: 50 mg, 100 mg.

Dosage: 50 mg twice daily before breakfast and at bedtime, increasing if necessary to 100 mg twice daily in the majority, and in a few cases to 200 mg twice daily.

The drug has no advantages over propranolol except in patients with mild chronic bronchitis; if beta-blockers are deemed necessary to control angina, metoprolol up to 100 mg twice daily is safer than an equivalent dose of propranolol. The drug's effectiveness may be affected by smoking.

## Nadolol

Supplied: Tablets: 40 mg, 80 mg, 120 mg, and 160 mg.

Dosage: 40 to 160 mg only *once* daily.

As with atenolol, food makes no difference to absorption and smoking does not alter effectiveness. After a few days or weeks at 40 mg daily, the drug is increased to 80 mg and in some patients to 160 mg daily. I have rarely found the need to increase the dose to the usual recommended maximum of 240 mg per day. The reason for this may be as follows: This drug, as well as atenolol, is eliminated from the body by the kidney. Many patients over age sixty have some degree of renal dysfunction and the drug is not eliminated quickly from the body. Drug accumulation may occur and cause a greater slowing of the pulse than expected. Therefore, patients over age sixty should be treated with small doses, e.g., 40 to 160 mg daily. If kidney failure is present, 40 mg every other day may be enough but in any case, your doctor's advice is necessary.

## Propranolol

Supplied: Tablets: 10 mg, 20 mg, 40 mg, 80 mg.
Dosage: 20 mg three times daily *before meals,* increasing slowly, under the supervision of your doctor, to 120 mg daily. After several weeks, a long-acting capsule of 80 mg or 160 mg of propranolol may be preferable. A dose of less than 80 mg daily is usually of no value since it takes more than this amount of the beta-blocker to block the effects of adrenaline and noradrenaline. Most patients with angina should receive 160 to 240 mg before adding a calcium antagonist or an oral nitrate. As emphasized, smoking decreases the effectiveness of propranolol.

## Calcium Antagonists

A new type of drug treatment for angina emerged in the early 1980s and has now become established as safe and effective medication for the treatment of angina.

Three calcium antagonists, diltiazem, nifedipine, and verapamil, have been approved for use in the United States and Canada. The Europeans and Japanese had experience with these drugs some five years earlier. The impact of these drugs has been such that some experts in cardiology have referred to calcium antagonists as the wonder drugs of the 1980s. They have found a place in the treatment of high blood pressure and in patients with severe palpitations (paroxysmal atrial tachycardia).

### How Do Calcium Antagonists Work?

Normally, the muscle present in the heart and walls of arteries contracts under the influence of a movement of calcium into the cells. Normally calcium is transported from the exterior to the interior of cells through a system of tubules called slow calcium channels. Calcium reaches the interior of muscle cells and interacts with specialized proteins in the muscle, which then contract. Dr. A. Fleckenstein of Germany has shown that this group of drugs block the slow calcium channels[11]; this action prevents calcium influx into the cell, thereby causing relaxation of the muscle of the heart and arteries. Various experts call the group of drugs calcium channel blockers, calcium entry blockers, slow channel blockers, or calcium antagonists. I prefer the term "calcium antagonist" since it is the one originally used by Fleckenstein and by the majority of experts as well, and the drugs have actions other than that of blocking calcium channels. Although the three mentioned drugs are grouped as calcium antagonists, their actions and side effects are as different as night and day. Available calcium antagonists and their doses are given in Table 11-1.

### Table 11-1 AVAILABLE CALCIUM ANTAGONISTS

| PREPARATION | TRADE NAME | SUPPLIED | DOSAGE |
| --- | --- | --- | --- |
| Nifedipine | Adalat | capsules | 10 mg t.i.d. |
| | Procardia | 5 mg | 3-30 days, then |
| | | 10 mg | 60 mg daily |
| | Adalat | tablets | 80 mg maximum |
| | Retard | 20 mg | |
| Verapamil | Isoptin | | |
| | Cordilox | tablets | |
| | | 40 mg (UK) | |
| | Cardimil | 80 mg | 80 mg t.i.d. |
| | Calan | 120 mg | 3-30 days, |
| | Isoptine | | 480 mg maximum |
| | Isoptino | ampoules | |
| | Manidon | 5 mg/2 ml | |
| | Vasolan | | 2-10 mg intravenously |
| | | | over 1-2 min. |
| Diltiazem | Cardizem | tablets | |
| | Anginyl | 30 mg | 60 mg q.i.d. |
| | Herbesser | 60 mg | 360 mg maximum |
| | Dilzem | | |
| | Masdil | | |

t.i.d.—three times daily
q.i.d.—four times daily

## Nifedipine

Supplied and dosage: See Table 11-1.
Indications

Nifedipine is of value in the treatment of:

1.  Variant angina (coronary artery spasm). All three available calcium antagonists—nifedipine, verapamil, and diltiazem—are equally effective in this rare condition.
2.  Stable angina pectoris in the following situations:
a.  If beta-blockers are contraindicated.
b.  In patients for whom beta-blockers at adequate doses achieve only slight relief or result in intolerable side effects. It is wise to discontinue beta-blockers slowly, replacing them with nifedipine or another calcium antagonist.
c.  If the response to adequate doses of beta-blockers is good but not completely effective. The addition of nifedipine is likely to result in further significant improvement.
3.  Unstable angina.
    Nifedipine is extremely valuable in the treatment of patients with unstable angina. The drug can be used alone but it is more efficient when combined with a beta-blocker. In an open trial, the combination of nifedipine and a beta-blocker has been shown to have a beneficial effect in patients with unstable angina.
4.  Angina complicated by heart failure or a left ventricular aneurysm or in individuals with peripheral vascular disease in which beta-blockers are contraindicated.
5.  Hypertension of all grades. The drug is superior to verapamil and diltiazem in patients with moderate or severe high blood pressure.
6.  Congestive heart failure. Nifedipine reduces the resistance against which the heart must pump; therefore, it reduces the workload of the heart and this helps patients with congestive heart failure. The drug may produce a beneficial effect in selective causes of heart failure if given with digoxin and a water pill (diuretic). In my experience, a dosage range in chronic heart failure of 10 mg three times daily to a maximum of 60 mg daily is of value.

7. Very cold fingers (Raynaud's phenomenon) and esophageal spasm.

## Actions, Advice and Adverse Effects

Nifedipine strongly blocks the slow calcium channels and
causes intense dilatation of arteries. The drug, therefore, dilates the coronary arteries and the arteries of the limbs and
elsewhere. This action causes a fall in the resistance in the
arteries, blood pressure falls, and the work of the heart is reduced. By causing less work for the heart, along with dilation of
the coronary arteries, the pain of angina is relieved. The drug
has no effect on the electrical system of the heart, and it is safe
in patients with electrical disturbances. The drug does not
cause a decrease in the contraction of heart muscle and can be
used in patients with heart failure. In fact the drug is commonly
used in the treatment of heart failure to reduce the workload
of the heart. This is accomplished by the dilation of arteries and
the reduction of the resistance against which the heart must
pump. In contrast, verapamil does not cause such intense arterial dilatation, but it does cause the heart muscle to reduce its
strength of contraction and consequently the drug can cause
heart failure. Diltiazem has similar effects to verapamil and
rarely precipitates heart failure or electrical disturbances. Because of these actions, nifedipine can be safely combined with a
beta-blocker, whereas, verapamil cannot be combined with a
beta-blocker except in patients with normal heart muscle function and a normal electrical conduction system. Diltiazem has
to be used with care when combined with a beta-blocker.
Nifedipine only rarely causes a problem when combined with a
beta-blocker.

There are no absolute contraindications to the use of
nifedipine. Dizziness occurs in some 3 to 12 percent of patients, and the drug must therefore be introduced slowly at a
dose of 10 mg twice daily for one to two days and then three
times daily as tolerated. If dizziness occurs, the drug is reduced. Dizziness can be made worse when nifedipine is combined with oral nitrates or nitrate preparations placed on the

skin or drugs that lower blood pressure. Edema of the legs occurs in about 5 percent of patients, but this does not indicate heart failure. It is due to dilatation of capillaries in the legs. Headaches and a throbbing sensation in the head can be distressing and occurs in some 5 to 10 percent of patients, and occasionally the drug has to be discontinued. However, patients must realize that the throbbing is not due to an increase in blood pressure but to dilation of the arteries in the scalp. The action is similar to a tablet of nitroglycerin put under the tongue. The headaches or throbbing become less severe after a few weeks of treatment, and the majority of patients can tolerate nifedipine at the dose of 60 to 80 mg daily. As the drug has such an important anti-anginal effect and no major side effects, patients are well advised to give the drug a fair trial even if it means reducing doses for a few weeks until the drug is tolerated. Mild flushing and burning in the scalp and head and occasional indigestion do occur. However, the drug does not produce or exacerbate stomach ulcers. Approximately 5 to 10 percent of patients discontinue the drug because of these minor yet distressing side effects.

Note that it is relatively safe to combine nifedipine with beta-blockers, but it is necessary to select patients carefully when verapamil or diltiazem are added to a beta-blocker because of the tendency for these agents to exacerbate very slow heart rate or heart failure. This complication is much worse with verapamil. I must reemphasize that all three calcium antagonists produce severe lowering of blood pressure. Care is therefore necessary when adding these medications to nitrates, beta-blockers, diuretics, or other drugs that cause a lowering of blood pressure.

### Verapamil

Supplied and dosage: See Table 11-1.
Indications

1.  Variant angina (coronary artery spasm), which is rare.
2.  Chronic stable angina pectoris not responsive to beta-blockers, in which case verapamil is an effective alternative.

3.  Stable angina pectoris, in combination with a beta-blocker in selected cases only. It is advisable to reduce the dose of beta-blocker when verapamil is added. I personally do not recommend the combination of verapamil with a beta-blocker because of the definite increase in the incidence of heart failure that this combination can produce.

4.  Severe palpitations (paroxysmal atrial tachycardia). Verapamil given intravenously in the emergency room is very effective and restores the heart rhythm to normal.

## Actions, Advice and Adverse Effects

Verapamil is a moderately potent vasodilator; however, the vasodilation of arteries is much less conspicuous than that seen with nifedipine. Verapamil causes a decrease in the contraction of heart muscle. This action can produce heart failure.

The drug blocks the electrical impulses to the atrioventricular node that connects the atrium to the ventricle. This action is beneficial because it stops the episodes of paroxysmal atrial tachycardia, as mentioned earlier.

Side effects include constipation, which may be distressing especially in the elderly. In the female, secretion of milk from the breasts (galactorrhea) and a minor degree of liver disturbance may rarely occur.

Verapamil is contraindicated in patients with a very slow pulse rate, heart block, sick sinus syndrome, heart failure, an enlarged heart, or poor heart muscle function.

## Drug Interactions

1.  With beta-blockers: Oral administration of verapamil combined with beta-blockers should be used with caution and only in selective patients because both drugs cause decreased contraction of heart muscle. Verapamil should not be given as a quick intravenous injection to patients receiving beta-blockers. Therefore, it is advisable at all times to have a card with you that lists your

medications or to bring your medications to the emergency room. This will help your doctors and enable them to render treatment much more quickly and efficiently.

2. With digoxin: Verapamil can increase the level of digoxin in the blood, and when both drugs are used, the physician has to recheck levels of digoxin more frequently and may need to lower the dose of both drugs.

3. With amiodarone: This is a drug that is used for the treatment of serious forms of extra beats (ventricular tachycardia) and should not be combined with verapamil.

4. With tranquilizers: When combined with tranquilizers, the patient should be warned about the possible sedative effects. In this regard, nifedipine does not cause sedation when used along with tranquilizers.

5. There is some evidence that verapamil increases the effects of anticoagulants (warfarin), and care must be taken to have the blood checked more frequently.

### Diltiazem

Supplied and dosage: Given in Table 11-1. However, I must emphasize that the majority of patients appear to need 240 mg or more to get relief from angina; the safety of doses greater than 360 mg daily has not as yet become well established.

Indications are the same as those listed for verapamil except that the drug is not used in the treatment of paroxysmal tachycardia since its effect is very mild.

### Actions, Advice and Adverse Effects

Diltiazem has a similar action as verapamil except that it is not as powerful. Note that it has to be given four times daily, whereas nifedipine can be given three times daily or twice daily in a sustained release preparation. Verapamil is given three times daily, but when used for more than several weeks, it can be reduced to twice daily in many patients, and a one-a-day preparation is currently being tested. Therefore, diltiazem at four times daily presents a problem with compliance since patients are not very eager to take medications four times daily, and they often forget to do so. The drug causes headaches and dizziness, but these are said to be less than with nifedipine. Disorientation and occasional, reversible elevation of liver enzymes (transaminases) have been seen in some patients.

There are other minor side effects of calcium antagonists, but there is no point burdening the reader with extreme detail. I have tried to point out problems with side effects and interactions that are relevant and thus protect the individual on this type of medication. Other calcium antagonists are being tested and will appear on the market by the end of the 1980s. I use diltiazem when there are side effects caused by nifedipine and verapamil.

## CORONARY ARTERY BYPASS SURGERY

Dr. Rene Favoloro of Argentina performed the first coronary artery bypass in 1967 at the Cleveland Clinic. He used a vein from a patient's leg to bypass the obstruction in the coronary artery. Since that time more than 1.5 million bypass operations have been performed. In 1984, some 200,000 patients had the operation in North America. The procedure is a simple one: A vein from the patient's leg is removed and inserted into the aorta as it leaves the heart; the other end of the vein is joined to the coronary artery below the blockage. Blood then flows from the aorta through the vein graft beyond the blockage to the coronary artery and to the heart muscle (see Figure 11-1). When possible, surgeons prefer to use the internal mammary artery to bypass the blockage instead of using a vein graft.

### Indications

If angina is not adequately relieved by the combination of a beta-blocker and calcium antagonist and lifestyle is deemed unacceptable by the patient or the physician, coronary artery bypass surgery is usually recommended. The main aim of sur-

# Figure 11-1 Coronary Bypass Graft
**Blood flows from the aorta to a coronary artery bypassing the blockage.**

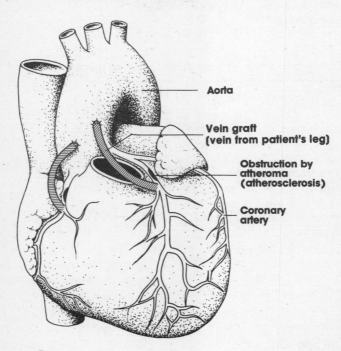

Aorta

Vein graft
(vein from patient's leg)

Obstruction by
atheroma
(atherosclerosis)

Coronary
artery

gery is therefore to relieve pain. The complete relief of pain is certainly most satisfying and this is achieved in 90 percent of patients, whereas drugs achieve this goal in very few. Drugs lessen the frequency of angina by about 60 percent in approximately 60 percent of patients treated. Such patients are satisfied and surgery is not indicated. Only about 20 percent get 90 percent relief. Thus about 20 percent of patients with angina are not satisfactorily controlled. Half of these are elderly or have illness that contraindicate surgical intervention. Thus, about 10 out of every 100 patients with "stable" angina are recommended to have coronary arteriography with a view to coronary bypass surgery. In some surgical centers, indications are broadened and many more patients are selected for surgery.

The majority of patients with unstable angina should be offered surgery if no major contraindication exists. Patients up to age seventy and, in some places, age seventy-five, are offered surgery. When surgery is done in 100 patients, the statistical outcome is as follows: The risk of dying during the surgery or within three days is 1 to 2 percent. Approximately 10 percent of patients have a heart attack during surgery, although it is usually silent and recovery is the rule. Approximately ninety patients get complete relief for two or more years. At the end of two years, fifteen to eighteen patients have obstruction of their grafts and some of these get a recurrence of the angina. Presently, with the addition of medication such as aspirin plus persantine, fewer grafts become blocked. After five years, about 70 percent of patients are still pain-free, lead active lives, and enjoy life to the fullest—a situation that does not materialize with the use of drug treatment in patients with frequent episodes of angina. Since the balloon crushing of atheroma (angioplasty) can be done only in a selected few, coronary bypass surgery will play a major role until about the turn of the century. The situation may change even earlier if laser therapy becomes beneficial and safe. Bypass surgery is simple to perform and there are few complications. Cardiac surgeons can be proud of this operation, which provides major relief for suffering and can prolong life in a selected few. I can visualize many successful operations using angioplasty and laser therapy during the next twenty years, but unless atherosclerosis is prevented, and this seems to be out of reach for the next fifty years, coronary artery bypass surgery will play a substantial role for longer than some experts predict. However, patients who have had surgery must understand that the other arteries and points in the coronary artery below the graft can develop further atherosclerosis since the operation does not cure the disease. In addition, a blood clot (coronary thrombosis) can form in any individual at any time without warning. Therefore, coronary bypass surgery does not prevent a second or third heart attack although it may prevent death in a few.

Prolongation of life may be achieved in the following types of patients:

1. Individuals who have severe narrowing of the left main coronary artery before it divides (see Figure 1-3). This is the anatomical lesion for which surgery is universally accepted and is fortunately rare.
2. Individuals who have triple vessel disease, that is, severe obstruction of the right coronary, the left anterior descending, and the circumflex arteries.
3. If the left anterior descending artery is blocked before its first branch, plus two other vessels have more than 80 percent obstructions.
4. Evidence of progressive disease based on clinical symptoms plus the results of the stress test.
a. Progressive angina, unstable angina.
b. Individuals who have a strongly positive stress test; the ECG shows severe oxygen lack for more than two minutes at low levels of exercise.
5. Angina with the presence of a left ventricular aneurysm.

Some clinical trials indicate that prolongation of life may be achieved in the above types of patients. I concur with these results although there are some reports to the contrary.

## Contraindications

Severe damage to the heart muscle as manifested by recurrent heart failure unresponsive to aggressive medical therapy is a major contraindication. Such patients are very short of breath and often have fluid in the lungs. Shortness of breath cannot be relieved by surgery, and the heart muscle is not strengthened. Several heart attacks cause large areas of scarring, and the scar tissue is very weak. Scar tissue is dead and not supplied with blood; therefore, a bypass graft does not feed blood to that area. However, heart failure in the presence of an acute heart attack that clears within the first seven days is not a contraindication to bypass surgery several months later.

Maintenance medications that are given after coronary bypass surgery include: a combination of 325 mg of aspirin (coated) three times daily and 50 to 75 mg of dipyridamole (Persantine) three times daily for two years to prevent blockage of the graft. Treatment beyond two years depends on individual surgeons.

Drugs such as beta-blockers, oral nitrates, and calcium antagonists are not usually required except in a few patients if angina recurs.

Patients are strongly advised not to recommence smoking. They are encouraged to engage in an exercise program and maintain a low-cholesterol–low-saturated-fat diet. The blood pressure should be checked every four months to be sure that it is not elevated since this may aggravate the problems of blockage in the graft.

It is important to understand that atherosclerotic disease is not cured by surgery. Coronary thrombosis can still occur. The vein graft can develop atherosclerosis over a period of five to ten years as veins are not usually subjected to the blood pressure found in arteries. The average pressure found within veins is normally about 5 to 7 mm Hg as compared to the normal pressure in arteries of about 110 to 150 mm Hg. One study showed that ten years post surgery, more than half of the grafts were narrowed or blocked—particularly in individuals with hypertension and increased cholesterol levels.[12]

## CORONARY ANGIOPLASTY

This new method of treatment of coronary heart disease is available in most major centers in North America. The first successful coronary angioplasty was performed by Dr. Gruntzig in Zurich in 1977; since then over 80,000 patients have been treated in North America and Europe. I must emphasize that it is a temporary measure. The obstructive plaque of atheroma is crushed at one point in one coronary artery. Atherosclerosis usually affects several segments of the coronary arteries, and as the disease process advances, every effort must be made to halt its progress.

The individual must try to control all risk factors—smoking must be discontinued; blood pressure must be kept within normal limits; stress must be alleviated; cholesterol should be monitored to run less than 200 mg/dL and at most 220 mg/dL, and diet plus or minus drug therapy may be necessary to achieve this goal. Beta-blockers and drugs to prevent thrombosis and restenosis may also be required after a successful coronary angioplasty.

## Indications

All patients are potential surgical candidates. Patients with severe angina who do not respond to medical therapy are candidates for angioplasty, if they have any of the following:

1. One coronary artery nearly completely obstructed (greater than 75 percent) by a discreet, preferably noncalcified plaque of atheroma. Patients with symptoms for less than six months with obstruction of the left anterior descending artery or right coronary artery before the artery gives off the first branch are the most ideal candidates.

2. During 1980 to 1983, indications were restricted to single vessel disease as outlined in indication 1. With increased experience and now steerable catheter systems, the indications have broadened. More difficult obstructions are undertaken by experts in some centers. Success is less likely to occur in patients with obstruction in the circumflex artery or at lower points (distal) in the coronary arteries, where there are irregular bends or turns.

3. Patients with acute heart attacks may have the clot dissolved by drugs such as streptokinase or tissue type plasminogen activator and then undergo coronary angioplasty to crush the plaque of atheroma that often lies beneath the clot.

## Contraindications

1. A coronary artery bypass surgical team is not available.
2. A totally blocked artery cannot be cleared because the catheter cannot be positioned.
3. Disease of the left main coronary artery before it divides into the anterior descending and circumflex branches presents too great a risk.
4. Severe atherosclerosis exists in all three vessels, although this is a relative contraindication.
5. The obstruction is in the terminal part of the artery and it cannot be reached by the balloon catheter.

In more than 50 percent of individuals with coronary heart disease, the obstruction in the artery is such that coronary angioplasty cannot be done. It is estimated that about 25 percent of patients who have angina and are suitable for coronary artery bypass surgery are candidates for coronary angioplasty.

## Technique for Cardiac Catheterization Arteriography and Coronary Angioplasty

The procedure is carried out in a cardiac catheterization laboratory under sterile conditions. The most common sites for inserting the wire or hollow plastic catheter are in the femoral artery located in the groin, the artery in the arm at the elbow, or, rarely, in the neck. These sites are preferred because the blood vessels are large and close to the skin surface.

The pulsation of the artery is easily felt and the skin is anesthetized with a local injection of anesthetic. When the skin is frozen and painless, a needle followed by thin wires is used to introduce the catheter into the artery. The catheter is then guided into the aorta and then into the cavity of the left ventricle. The catheter position is visualized at all times with the aid of an X-ray fluoroscope, which shows the catheter on a screen. This procedure is called cardiac catheterization. The same technique is utilized for performing coronary arteriography (angiograms) or for studying the heart valves and pressures inside the heart chambers. However, for the technique of coronary angioplasty, a specialized catheter is used. It has a double lumen and a small inflatable balloon at the tip (Figure 11-2). The length of the balloon is about 2.5 cm and the inflated diameter is 2 to 4 mm. The catheter is guided into the appropriate coronary artery to the obstruction previously visualized by coronary arteriography. During coronary arteriography, dye that looks white on X-ray film (radio-opaque) is injected into a catheter positioned selectively in the right and the left coronary arteries.

All patients undergoing coronary angioplasty or coronary artery bypass surgery must have coronary arteriography to show the cardiologist or surgeon the exact site of blockage by a plaque of atheroma. Arteriography can be done several hours or several months prior to such further procedures.

The procedure, percutaneous transluminal coronary angioplasty (PTCA), is so named because the instrument is passed through the skin (percutaneous) and then through the lumen of the artery (transluminal) into the coronary artery, which is molded into shape (angioplasty). The balloon-tipped catheter is positioned next to the plaque of atheroma in the artery. The balloon is inflated for a duration of thirty to sixty seconds and the plaque is squashed by the pressure. The narrowed artery becomes dilated due to splitting (dissection) of the plaque and overstretching of the middle wall (media) of the artery. Transient chest pain may occur during the inflation but this is quickly relieved. Several inflations may be necessary to accomplish dilation of the artery. The balloon is then deflated and dye is injected to visualize if adequate dilation and flow of blood has been achieved.

Following the angioplasty, the patient is monitored in the coronary care unit for twenty-four to forty-eight hours. The total hospital stay is usually three days. Most centers give

# Figure 11-2 Coronary Angioplasty

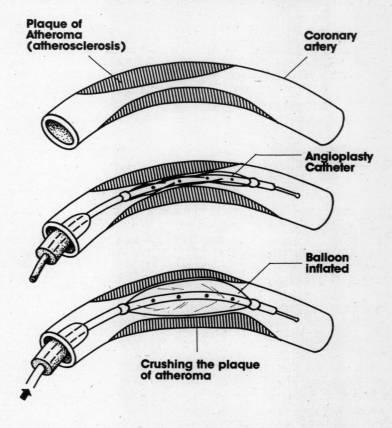

Plaque of
Atheroma
(atherosclerosis)

Coronary
artery

Angioplasty
Catheter

Balloon
inflated

Crushing the plaque
of atheroma

patients a combination of 325 mg aspirin and 50 to 75 mg dipyridamole three times daily for six to twelve months in an attempt to prevent platelet adhesions to the damaged surface and thus prevent restenosis (narrowing) of the artery.

## Outcome

Successful reopening of the artery is achieved in 70 to 90 percent of cases, and with improved blood flow, angina improves.[13] The majority of patients return to work seven to fourteen days later and have no recurrence of the angina for at least six months. The major early complications include the following: Death occurs in 1 percent of cases. A heart attack occurs in 5 percent of cases, because the crushing and splitting of the plaque of atheroma exposes cells and substances that promote blood clotting. Emergency surgery is necessary in about 5 to 7 percent of cases, and the emergency operation has a 4 to 5 percent mortality.[14] Prolonged chest pain occurs in about 7 percent of cases. In about 25 percent, it is not possible to pass the catheter through the narrowed area. In about 10 percent, the dilation cannot be accomplished because the plaques are calcified and rock-hard.

These complications approach those of coronary artery by-pass surgery.[13] The chief late complication at the site of angioplasty is further narrowing of the artery (restenosis), in approximately 33 percent of cases. Fortunately, these narrowings can be dilated more easily on the second procedure than on the first.[14] Restenosis occurs in 20 to 35 percent of patients within six months of the procedure, and such patients have a return of their chest pain.

Long-term results are not yet available. The National Heart, Lung and Blood Institute's Registry Data reveals that of the 1,418 patients filed at one year, 73 (2.7 percent) had died, 8.5 percent had repeat coronary angioplasty, and 33 percent had coronary artery bypass surgery.[13] At three years, only 36 percent of those followed were symptom-free. There is no evidence to suggest that the procedure prolongs life. I must reemphasize that coronary angioplasty is not in competition with coronary artery bypass surgery. Approximately 70 percent of individuals cannot have coronary angioplasty and must have coronary artery bypass surgery. However, coronary angioplasty is much cheaper, the hospital stay is only three days, and return to work is within one to two weeks. Once the complication of restenosis is overcome and five- to ten-year follow-up is available, the role of coronary angioplasty may be expanded.

I will summarize the important statistics that enable both physician and patient to make decisions. Twenty-five percent of patients who require coronary bypass surgery are suitable candidates for coronary angioplasty. If 100 of these patients are selected, 33 percent cannot be dilated because the catheters cannot get through to the lesion or cannot crush it because it is rock-hard. Of those who undergo angioplasty, 1 percent die, 5 percent have a heart attack within twenty-four hours, 5 percent require emergency surgery, and 85 percent have a successful result, are pain-free, and able to do much more work. Thirty-three percent are restenose within six months and more than half of these can be redilated. Approximately 33 percent usually require coronary artery bypass surgery within the next year.

## IS LASER THERAPY REALLY COMING?

Currently many type of lasers are being tested. Lasers are capable of getting rid of plaques of atheroma in experimental animals. In animals the coronary artery atheroma can be dissolved in the majority; however, perforation of the artery is common. In human cadaver experiments obstruction by atheroma can be removed. Various experiments have been done to show that the debris released is not potentially harmful.

In man, plaques of atheroma in the femoral artery in the thigh have been successfully dissolved by laser, resulting in relief of pain in the legs during walking. A few centers are doing some experimental work on coronary artery obstruction. The laser is passed down a catheter to reach the obstruction in the coronary artery. The laser is fired, dissolves the blockage, and blood flow is restored to the previously blocked artery. Perforation of the artery is the major hazard, but if we can fly to the moon, I am sure we will soon learn to operate the most beneficial type of laser. Advantages are such that by 1990 treatment in man should be feasible. It is very likely that the balloon coronary angioplasty will be replaced during the 1990s by laser coronary angioplasty.

# CHAPTER 12

# CARDIOPULMONARY RESUSCITATION (CPR)

Perhaps you may happen to be near someone who falls to the ground and stops breathing. You may be alone or someone summons you to help. *Can you help?* If you have never seen CPR done or tried to do it, I dare say it will not be easy to detect if the heart has stopped, give mouth-to-mouth resuscitation, and compress the victim's chest. Thus it is wise for all individuals to attend a practical course in CPR or at least read and practice the drill until it becomes automatic. The technique is really quite simple. However, you must realize that when you assist an individual, you are really trying to get oxygen to the brain to keep it alive until expert help arrives. I have summarized the points to assist you when faced with an individual who has "dropped dead" in your presence so that you may render some valuable assistance.

Patients may lose consciousness and fall over because of several reasons. For example:

1. A simple faint. The patient has a pulse, does not stop breathing, and there is no shaking of the limbs. Simply keeping the head down, preferably with the individual lying flat, and raising the legs up in the air above the patient's hips will cause blood to flow from the legs. Over a thirty-second to one-minute period, the individual will recover completely.

2. A seizure (epilepsy). The patient's limbs show typical movements that are jerky, the limbs get rigid, and

there is a combination of rigidity and jerking of one or more limbs. The patient is breathing but saliva and foam bubble from the mouth; some individuals pass urine or stools; recovery is the norm.

3.  A stroke. During a stroke, circulation to part of the brain is cut off because of a blood clot in an artery in the brain. Strokes usually occur in individuals over age sixty. It is rare for the patient to fall suddenly to the floor without some warning. The patient will have a pulse, and breathing will be present. Unlike with a simple faint, elevating the limbs, which should be tried, is not successful over a period of one to two minutes. There is no reason to do CPR since the heartbeat, circulation, and respirations still exist.

4.  Cardiac arrest. During a cardiac arrest, the heart stops beating completely and is at a standstill (asystole) in about 25 percent of individuals. In about 75 percent, the cardiac arrest is due to ventricular fibrillation, during which the heart muscle does not contract, but quivers. During ventricular fibrillation, there is no effective heart contraction, and blood is not pumped to the brain or other parts of the body. Ventricular fibrillation can be treated by an electrical shock, which defibrillates the heart and replaces the ventricular fibrillation with a normal heartbeat. In standstill or asystole, there is no electrical current in the heart and the shock is of no value. In a few of these cases, the heart may commence beating on its own; the condition is called a Stokes-Adams attack, derived from the doctors who first described it. The condition, which is described in Chapter 15, is extremely rare. The majority of patients with asystole perish because the heart attack is very large. A few can be saved by the insertion of a pacemaker if the attack is in the hospital.

It is wise for a family member of a heart patient to have knowledge of CPR. This certainly reassures the patient that possibly something can be done. The knowledgeable individual also feels some sense of confidence, which promotes hope. You must realize that CPR is only a temporary measure. The aim is to get blood containing a fresh supply of oxygen to the brain.

Therefore, you need to breathe enough air into the patient's lung, then compress the chest to cause the nonbeating heart to expel blood into the arteries, thus producing a circulation of the blood to the brain. The rare patient may be revived and the heart beats spontaneously. However, in the majority with asystole, nothing can be done outside of a hospital, and in those with ventricular fibrillation, death will occur unless the heart is defibrillated. Therefore, the $64,000 question is, Does the ambulance have a portable defibrillator and a team that can defibrillate the patient? If this is present, then there is hope. In any event, I will summarize the important principles and methods of CPR since they are simple to apply. You should also contact your local chapter of the American Heart Association or the Red Cross to ascertain where CPR courses are held.

## RECOGNITION OF CARDIAC ARREST

1. The patient is *unconscious* and has a deathlike appearance.
2. The patient is *not breathing*. You should verify this.
3. There is *no pulse*. Check for a pulse by feeling the carotid artery in the neck. The right carotid artery is felt from about one inch from the angle of the jaw. Place your right index finger in a straight line next to (parallel with) the windpipe (trachea) so that the entire length of the first finger pad is overlying the skin. The tip of the index finger should be approximately opposite the Adam's apple. You can also start by feeling the most prominent part of the Adam's apple with the tip of the index finger, then slide the finger outward to reach the groove between the hard cartilage of the windpipe and the muscle of the neck. The carotid artery lies only a few millimeters under the skin and the pulsation is easily felt. Practice feeling this pulse so that you can find it in a hurry, taking no more than ten seconds. Therefore, within thirty seconds you should have arrived at a conclusion that a cardiac arrest has occurred. Speed of diagnosis is critical. Within three

to four minutes of cardiac arrest, irreversible brain damage can occur because of lack of oxygen. The resuscitation procedures listed below follow the recommendations of the American Heart Association.[15]

Your intention is to provide basic life support until advanced life support in the form of expert technical help arrives. Basic life support consists of:

1. The recognition of cardiac arrest.
2. The proper application of cardiopulmonary resuscitation to maintain life until advanced life support is available.

## THE A-B-C STEPS OF CPR

The A-B-C steps of CPR should be commenced immediately. Quickly turn the victim flat on the back on a hard surface (preferably the floor).

**A: Airway.** Open the airway by placing one hand under the victim's neck close to the head and the other hand on the forehead, and tilt the victim's head backward as far as possible. The eyes then look directly upward. The head must be maintained in this position at all times (see Figure 12-1).[16] This position ensures that the air passages remain open. Do not allow the chin to move toward the chest.

**B: Breathing.** Pinch the victim's nostrils closed. Then take a deep breath, make a tight seal over the victim's mouth with your mouth, and blow into the victim's mouth. Ventilate the victim rapidly four times without allowing his or her lungs to deflate completely between the breaths. At this point, check for the carotid pulse using the hand that was behind the victim's neck.

**C: Circulation.** If no pulse is present, begin compressing the external chest. Place the heel of one hand over the lower half of the breastbone but at least one inch (two finger-breadths) away from the end of the breastbone (xiphoid process). Position the heel of the second hand on the top of the first. *Keep the fingers off the rib cage* (Figure 12-1). If the hands are applied

# Figure 12-1 The ABC of cardiopulmonary resuscitation

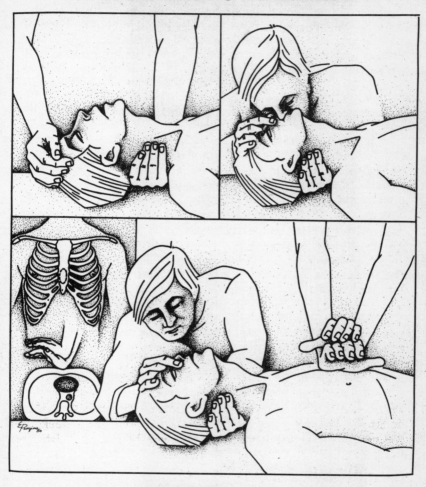

A The airway is opened.
B Breathing: The victim's nostrils are pinched closed and the rescuer breathes into the victim's mouth.
C Circulation: If no pulse is present, external chest compression is instituted.

too high, ineffective chest compression may result, and fracture of the ribs may occur. Keep the arms straight at the elbow (locked elbows) and apply pressure as vertically as possible. Your shoulders should be directly above the victim's breast-bone. Chest compressions are thus easily carried out by forceful movements of the shoulders and back, so the maneuver is less tiring. Depress the breastbone 1½ to 2 inches toward the spine, and maintain a 50% compression–50% relaxation cycle.

If there is only a *single* rescuer, use fifteen compressions to two ventilations.

If there are *two* rescuers, use five compressions to one ventilation.

*CPR should never be interrupted for more than five seconds.* It should be continued until skilled help arrives.

Note that the victim's mouth should be almost completely closed. However, depress the lower lip a bit so that the mouth remains slightly opened. If dentures cannot be managed in place, remove them after first giving the very important first four breaths. If you wish, you can place a clean gauze or folded handkerchief over the patient's mouth and nose. Rescuers can rarely contract tuberculosis or hepatitis from victims. Special airways are available but they are never handy when desperately required. However, in the case of family members, infection is never a consideration.

You must see the chest rise and fall. There is no logical reason at the commencement of CPR to first look for foreign bodies or vomitus before giving the first four breaths. If the first four breaths meet with resistance and the chest fails to rise when you breathe air into the patient's mouth, make sure that the airway is properly opened by the head tilt and that the seal around the mouth is air-tight, then clear the airway with your fingers if necessary. The fact that the patient suddenly dropped to the ground and the immediate circumstances—for example, without choking while eating—are sufficient to persuade you not to waste time searching for meat or vomitus. The maneuvers used for clearing foreign bodies, in particular, the very useful Heimlich maneuver, are not appropriate for cardiac arrest and thus not described here.

## The Precordial Thump

The public is advised not to use the precordial thump. The thump is used when the patient is attached to a cardiac monitor and the continuous electrocardiograph is recorded. If a doctor or nurse sees ventricular fibrillation or ventricular tachycardia (another abnormal fast heart rhythm), the precordial thump is then immediately carried out. The thump is likely to restore normal heart rhythm only if delivered within thirty seconds of the onset of the two abnormal rhythms mentioned. The thump remains a controversial issue even in the indications outlined. Thus, many experts do not recommend its use even in the hospital setting.

You can do your part and learn CPR and encourage groups in your community to do the same. In cities where a rapid-response emergency care system is utilized in conjunction with citizens trained in CPR, countless lives have been saved.

The Belfast, Brighton, and Seattle services are well known, and their noble example has been followed by cities such as Cleveland, Dallas, Dayton, Houston, Jacksonville, Miami, St. Paul, and Washington, D.C. Might not a telethon help this noble cause in other cities?

# PART III

# OTHER CARDIOVASCULAR DISEASES

# CHAPTER 13

# HYPERTENSION

Hypertension, commonly known as high blood pressure, is a problem suffered by more than 60 million people in North America. The results of high blood pressure often lead to early death or serious physical handicaps. There are generally very few symptoms associated with high blood pressure, and health complaints may not surface for five to twenty years, thus the term "the silent killer."

Blood pressure is the pressure exerted by the blood against the inner walls of the blood vessels, especially the arteries. The blood pressure changes from minute to minute and is influenced by many factors such as activity, age, health, emotional tension, and so on. With each heartbeat, about 70 milliliters of blood are ejected from the heart and propelled through approximately 100,000 kilometers of blood vessels. Constriction of the blood vessels (arteries) causes high blood pressure and greatly increases the work of the heart. Arteries are traumatized by high blood pressure and this increases the development of hardening of the arteries owing to plaques of atheroma (atherosclerosis). The heart may enlarge, arteries may become gradually blocked, and circulation to the heart muscle, the brain, and other organs may slowly become impaired until one day there will be an emergency situation such as a sudden heart attack or stroke. It is true that hypertension maims and kills millions through complications that are nearly all preventable.

Have your blood pressure checked. The onus is on you; you can save yourself from "the silent killer."

Clinical trials during the 1980s have revolutionized the

211

treatment of hypertension with and without drugs. Many familiar (old) drugs have been rendered obsolete because of safer and more effective alternatives. As there are so many antihypertensive drugs that both physicians and patients may become confused, I feel that up-to-date information, on the new medications in particular, may help to clarify and to simplify the treatment of hypertension.

If you have high blood pressure, safe and effective treatment is available either with nondrug programs or with a suitably selected drug. Drug selection is important and is discussed in some detail.

## WHAT IS BLOOD PRESSURE?

Hypertension is the medical term for high blood pressure and has nothing to do with being hyper, or excessive nervous tension. The heart pumps blood directly into blood vessels called arteries, which are like a series of pipes. The narrower the arteries, the greater the resistance or impedance to the flow of blood; therefore the heart must pump with greater force. The amount of force with which the blood is being pumped from the heart through the arteries is the blood pressure. The blood exerts pressure against the artery walls, thus the term "blood pressure." Everyone has blood pressure, and we will discuss later what is meant by high blood pressure. The pressure in the arteries when the heart contracts (systole) is called systolic blood pressure, usually this is less than 140 millimeters (mm) Hg (mercury). The pressure in the arteries when the heart is relaxed (diastole) is called diastolic pressure, and this is usually less than 90 mm Hg. Another way of looking at blood pressure is as follows: Each contraction of the heart causes blood to be pushed (propelled) through the arteries in the form of a pulse wave; thus the flow of blood in the arteries is pulsatile. A wave must have a crest and a trough. The crest is caused when the heart contracts (systole) and is the highest pressure or systolic blood pressure. The trough is caused when the heart relaxes (diastole), producing the lowest pressure or diastolic pressure.

The resistance in the arteries against which the heart must pump is called the total vascular resistance. If the total vascular resistance increases, blood pressure increases. This resistance is increased when the arteries are constricted by disease, drugs, or naturally occurring chemicals in the body such as adrenaline. The amount of blood expelled by the heart into the arteries in one minute is called the cardiac output and is about five liters per minute. Blood pressure is equal to the total vascular resistance multiplied by the cardiac output.

## MEASUREMENT OF BLOOD PRESSURE

The instrument used to measure blood pressure is called a sphygmomanometer. It measures the air pressure needed to raise a column of mercury (Hg). The instrument consists of an inflatable cuff connected to a small bulb-pump and a pressure gauge. By means of the inflatable cuff, which encircles the limb, air pressure within the cuff is balanced against the pressure in the artery (usually the brachial artery at the elbow); the pressure is estimated by means of a mercury or aneroid manometer. The mercury manometer is the most accurate pressure gauge. The aneroid gauge is frequently used instead of the mercury manometer since this is more compact and is convenient as a portable instrument but it should be calibrated twice yearly. I must point out that some electronic instruments may give falsely high diastolic readings, but manufacturers will improve to meet market demands.

The cuff size is of great importance. If the cuff is too small for the patient's arm, the blood pressure reading may be falsely high. In this case some moderately obese patients may be falsely classified as hypertensives if a normal cuff is used. A regular cuff may be used for arm circumference less than thirty-three centimeters. A large cuff, fifteen centimeters by thirty-three centimeters, should be used whenever the patient's mid–upper arm circumference exceeds thirty-three centimeters. The cuff must be applied snugly. To measure blood pressure, the cuff is wrapped around the arm about one inch above the elbow crease. Ask your doctor or nurse to show you how to take your own blood pressure. Occasionally both the radial pulse at the wrist and the brachial pulse at the elbow over which the stethoscope is placed are difficult to feel, and you may become frustrated with the attempt. Get your doctor to determine your systolic blood pressure using the stethoscope and also by palpation, ie., using his fingers on the pulse at the wrist. Have him or her write down your blood pressure and you should keep this recording.

**Step 1.** Remove restricted clothing from the arm to shoulder (no tight, rolled-up shirt sleeve).

**Step 2.** You should be lying or sitting comfortably. The forearm should rest on a comfortable support such as a table at near heart level. If the arm is not well supported, muscle contractions will falsely elevate the blood pressure.

**Step 3.** Apply the cuff so that the arrow ( ↓ ) or mark on the cuff is directly in line with the brachial artery (Figure 13-1). The arrow on the edge of the cuff is then approximately one inch above the point of application of the stethoscope.

**Step 4.** Feel the radial pulse at the wrist. Close the valve of the instrument and hold the bulb in the right hand between the palm and fingers. Squeeze the bulb rapidly and fully. Continue squeezing the bulb several times to pump air into the cuff. The air pressure will at some point stop the blood flow through the brachial and radial arteries. Rapid inflation avoids trapping of blood in the veins of the forearm. As the cuff is inflated the radial pulse at the wrist will disappear. Keep on pumping so that the manometer pressure is increased by another 20 to 30 mm Hg or to 200 mm Hg. Then gradually open the valve, decreasing the pressure slowly at a rate of about 2 mm per second until you can just feel the radial pulse. Note the reading in mm Hg. This is the systolic blood pressure by palpation. To obtain your blood pressure using a stethoscope: If your systolic blood pressure is usually 140 mm Hg, pump the cuff up to a pressure on the gauge of 170 then put the

# Figure 13-1. Measurement of Blood Pressure

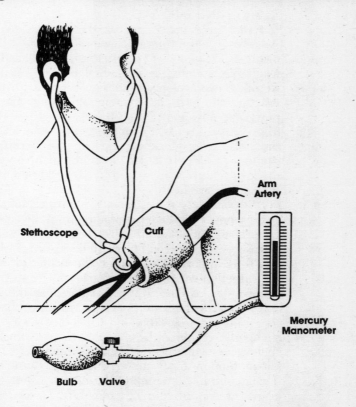

stethoscope on the brachial artery (position as indicated in Figure 13-1) then slowly release the air. Suddenly you will hear thudding sounds, which are impossible to miss if the room is quiet and the stethoscope earpieces are fitting snugly. The sounds are produced by the blood being pushed by each heartbeat through the artery previously blocked by the air pressure. The air pressure recorded by the gauge in mm Hg at which you first hear the sounds is the systolic blood pressure. These thudding sounds produced by blood movement and vessel vibrations are called Korotkoffs sounds, as described by Dr. Nicolai Korotkoff over seventy years ago. When you were inflating the cuff, the reason for asking you to pump the air about 20 to 30 mm above the systolic pressure is to pick up the rare case in which the stethoscope does not pick up the Korotkoff sounds early enough. However, in such cases if the air pressure is increased by 10 or 20 mm Hg, the sounds are heard.

**Step 5.** Further decrease the air pressure until all sounds just disappear and take the reading from the gauge as the diastolic blood pressure. Record, for example, as follows: "systolic 140, diastolic 80; or 140/80."

It is important to center the arrow on the cuff directly over the brachial artery. The stethoscope must be placed also directly over the artery. Your doctor can work out the line of the artery for you. The tendon of the biceps can be felt in the crook of the elbow and the artery is about one centimeter off-center, medial to the biceps tendon, i.e., nearer the body. Place the stethoscope in the crook of the elbow just to the inside of the middle of your forearm (Figure 13-1). It can be helpful to tape the stethoscope's diaphragm to the elbow if you are measuring your own blood pressure. If you wish to repeat the blood pressure reading, you must completely deflate the cuff and wait sixty seconds; otherwise congestion of blood in the veins of the arm can cause subsequent diastolic readings to be falsely high.

Occasionally it may be necessary to take blood pressure both in the lying and standing positions, especially if the patient is on medication. Some antihypertensive drugs cause the blood pressure to drop suddenly when the patient stands, and this is termed postural hypotension. In some patients over sixty-five years of age, markedly hardened vessels may require higher cuff pressures to stop the blood flow through the artery. This results in falsely high systolic pressure readings. This is one of the reasons why systolic hypertension in the elderly in the presence of a normal diastolic blood pressure is not often treated with drugs.

## HOW HIGH IS HIGH?

The World Health Organization and many experts agree that in individuals under age sixty-five, a systolic blood pressure above 160 and a diastolic blood pressure above 95 (160/95) is abnormal, and a blood pressure below 140/90 is normal. The intermediate range of borderline hypertension—systolic 140 to 160—is a controversial area. However, the Framingham Study and other studies indicate a significant increase in cardiovascular risk in individuals with a blood pressure in the borderline range. In the United States, an individual is considered to have high blood pressure if several readings exceed 140/90, especially if three consecutive readings are elevated. The risk at any level of hypertension including borderline hypertension is greatly increased by smoking or a high blood cholesterol. Mild hypertension is extremely common, and over a ten- to fifteen-year period increases the risk of stroke, heart attack, and heart failure. Clinical studies have documented that blacks develop organ damage (stroke or heart failure) much quicker than whites at the same level of hypertension.

Your blood pressure changes from minute to minute and is lowest during sleep, dropping as much as 10 to 30 mm Hg. It rises in the morning and usually becomes higher in the afternoon. This makes it necessary to measure the blood pressure several times during the day and to record the time of the measurement. An average of at least three readings is often taken by the doctor. Blood pressure increases to the adult level by age sixteen. The systolic blood pressure tends to increase slightly after age thirty. After age sixty-five, a greater increase often occurs, owing primarily to hardening of the arteries, and a falsely elevated pressure may be recorded.

I must emphasize, the division between high and normal is arbitrary and based mainly on the Framingham data, which shows that more cardiovascular diseases will appear in individuals with pressures exceeding 140/90. Hypertension is present in individuals under age 65 if three measurements taken at approximately the same time of day exceeds 140/90.

Hypertension is mild if the diastolic blood pressure is 91 to 105 or systolic pressure is 150 to 190. Hypertension is moderate if the diastolic is 106 to 114 or systolic greater than 200. Hypertension is severe if the diastolic is 115 to 130, regardless of the systolic pressure, and very severe if the diastolic is greater than 130 mm. The latter is termed malignant hypertension if the doctor finds swelling of the optic disc, hemorrhages in the eyes (retina), and kidney failure. Fortunately, such a situation is becoming very rare with the proper drug management of moderate and severe hypertension.

Prior to 1970, doctors believed that it was mainly the high diastolic blood pressure that was dangerous. However, an elevated systolic blood pressure is as important as an elevated diastolic pressure. Such elevations in systolic blood pressure increases the risk of heart failure or stroke. The danger of heart failure is considerably increased if the patient has had a previous heart attack or heart failure, or has an enlarged heart.

The heart rate multiplied by the systolic blood pressure is termed the heart rate pressure product, and this product determines the oxygen requirement of the heart muscle. Elevation of the systolic blood pressure is just as bad as elevation of the diastolic in the range 95 to 110 mm. Elevation of either systolic or diastolic is important, but the combined elevation is more common and further increases the risks. Drugs that decrease both the blood pressure and the heart rate are more effective in decreasing the oxygen requirement of the heart muscle. As we will see later, the beta-blocking drugs play a very important role in the drug treatment of hypertension because of the aforementioned effects.

# CAUSES OF HYPERTENSION

## Primary (essential) Hypertension

In the majority of cases of hypertension, no detectable underlying disease is present. There are several theories as to why the blood pressure may be increased, but no disease of organs or tissues is present. This type of hypertension is called primary to distinguish it from secondary hypertension, for which causes can be defined with certainty.

Primary hypertension has always been referred to as essential hypertension. The word "essential" was used because it was believed that higher pressures were needed to pump blood through arteries that were narrowed for some unknown reason. The use of the word has been so ingrained that it cannot be easily removed.

## Secondary Hypertension

In only 5 to 10 percent of all hypertensive patients can an underlying cause be defined. The most common causes include (1) kidney diseases, (2) coarctation of the aorta, (3) endocrine (hormonal) diseases, and (4) birth control pills.

1.  Kidney diseases include infections such as pyelonephritis, nephritis (Bright's Disease), congenital cysts in the kidney (congenital polycystic kidney), and blockage of the artery that feeds the kidney with blood (renal artery stenosis). These conditions are easy to exclude by the physician's taking your history and examining

the kidneys and urine and performing special X-rays such as an intravenous pyelogram (IVP) and arteriograms of the kidneys. The renal causes of hypertension occur in all age groups: children may get nephritis; blockage of the renal arteries may occur owing to thickening of the muscular wall of the artery, especially in young women; or in the elderly, blockage may be caused by atherosclerotic plaques.

2.  Coarctation of the aorta is a severe constriction of the large artery (aorta) that leaves the heart (Figure 1-2). Although present from birth, the condition may not cause symptoms and may go undetected into childhood or adult life. This condition is easy to exclude. The blood pressure is low in the legs and the pulses to the legs (femoral felt in the groin) are weak and delayed compared with the pulses in the upper limbs. Chest X-rays and arteriograms can confirm the diagnosis. In the majority of cases the condition is easily corrected by surgery.

3.  Endocrine (hormonal). This is usually due to an increase in hormone secretions from the adrenal glands. The adrenal glands lie on the upper pole of each kidney. The following are diseases of the adrenal glands.

a.  Cushing's Syndrome. Excess cortisone and its derivatives are secreted from the outer part (cortex) of the gland and cause hypertension. There is a redistribution of fat and a typical moon face, with obesity of the trunk; the arms and legs are relatively thin and the thigh muscles often become weak. Fortunately, surgery can produce a cure.

b.  Hyperaldosteronism, or Conn's Syndrome. This is due to a small benign tumor that secretes aldosterone. This hormone causes a retention of salt and water in the body and an excretion of potassium in the urine. Thus, the serum potassium is low. The condition is rare and when diagnosed can be cured surgically.

c.  Pheochromocytoma. The center of the gland (medulla) produces adrenaline (epinephrine) and noradrenaline (norepinephrine). A tumor of this area causes excessive secretions and produces very severe hypertension. Fortunately, the condition is rare, about 0.1 percent of all hypertensives. The condition is important, however, since it is life-threatening, but when diagnosed, is surgically correctable. The features are often typical. In about 50 percent of cases, the blood pressure is relatively constant, and in the other 50 percent, the blood pressure fluctuates with paroxysms of severe hypertension occurring daily, weekly, or monthly. The patient is quite well between episodes. During episodes symptoms include very severe, intolerable, throbbing headaches; profuse sweating and palpitations; fear of impending doom; seizure-like activity or psychoneurotic spells; weight loss; and postural hypotension (the blood pressure is very high, but may fall on standing). The blood pressure may be normal for several days or months and then suddenly rises to levels of 190 to 300 systolic and 100 to 160 diastolic. Fortunately, the condition is easy to exclude by urine test for adrenaline, noradrenaline, and breakdown products called vanillylmandelic acid (VMA) and metanephrines. A computerized tomographic scan (CT scan of the adrenals) will diagnose virtually all cases. However, doctors cannot run these tests on all of the 60 million hypertensives in North America. Therefore, the physician and patient should be alerted by such symptoms and initiate screening tests when warranted. Another important clue to the diagnosis is a failure to respond to the usual antihypertensive drugs or a marked increase in blood pressure that may be provoked by certain drugs. For example, the patient's blood pressure may increase with certain medications such as nasal decongestants containing adrenaline-like compounds, antihypertensive agents such as methyldopa, and opiates such as morphine and demerol.

Increased activity of the thyroid (hyperthyroidism, thyrotoxicosis) occasionally causes mild systolic hypertension.

4. Birth control pills. Estrogen-containing oral contraceptive pills are an increasing cause of mild hypertension in young women. About 5 percent of users develop hypertension. The hypertension is usually mild, but rarely, severe hypertension can occur, resulting in

kidney damage. On discontinuing the pill, the blood pressure returns to normal in the majority within six months. The increase in blood pressure described may be less with the newer low-dose estrogen contraceptive pill. The low-dose (0.3 to 0.625 mg) conjugated estrogen used to treat postmenopausal hot flashes very rarely cause a mild increase in blood pressure.

## MALIGNANT HYPERTENSION

This is a very serious condition. The diastolic blood pressure is usually greater than 130 for several hours or weeks. When such a diastolic blood pressure is associated with organ damage notably to the vessels in the eyes, kidneys, or brain, the diagnosis is confirmed. The blood pressure increases rapidly over days or weeks to dangerous levels, and the systolic may be as high as 250 to 300 and the diastolic 130 to 160. The retina of the eyes often show hemorrhages and edema of the optic disc. Small arteries are severely damaged; in particular the kidney vessels are damaged and leak red blood cells. The urine therefore contains numerous red cells (microscopic hematuria). The function of the kidney rapidly deteriorates and a brain hemorrhage may also occur. Life is threatened by this severe damage to the kidney, brain, eyes, and heart.

Fortunately, the condition is decreasing in incidence because of effective drug treatment of the moderate forms of hypertension. The reassuring news is that it is rare for a patient with the very common mild primary hypertension to develop malignant hypertension. The patient usually has moderate hypertension for a short period, blood pressure 200–250/105–120. In some cases the malignant phase is precipitated by kidney disease, such as nephritis, but rarely renal vascular hypertension (renal artery stenosis) or collagen disease such as scleroderma or pheochromocytoma. The malignant hypertension can be quickly brought under control by a range of effective drugs given intravenously. This form of hypertension cannot be treated without drugs. The blood pressure may be very high—250/150—yet headaches can be absent. Other causes of hypertension include brain tumors, bleeding around the surface of the brain from a ruptured artery (subarachnoid hemorrhage), spinal cord injuries, and the well-known hypertension of pregnancy.

## IS EXCESS SALT INTAKE THE CAUSE OF HIGH BLOOD PRESSURE

The hypothesis accepted by the majority of researchers is that an inherited defect causes the kidney to retain excess sodium (salt) in the body. If you have such an inherited defect and your diet contains a large amount of sodium, your kidneys will retain more sodium and water. A normal kidney that has no defect in handling sodium will put out in the urine any excess that you may add in the diet. The sodium and water retained by the kidney get into the blood and also into the cells of the artery wall, thereby increasing the tone of the artery wall. This means that the artery becomes constricted or tightened and increases the resistance against which the heart must pump, i.e., there is an increase in total vascular resistance and an increase in blood pressure (Figure 13-2).

You may understand the relationship between salt and hypertension if you look at the following example: If an individual is bleeding severely from a large cut or from the stomach or other body site, the blood pressure always falls, sometimes to very low levels such as 75/50. A transfusion of blood must be given quickly to increase the blood pressure, because at such a low level, not enough oxygen, glucose, and other nutrients will reach the brain, muscles of the heart, and other tissues of the body. However, blood is not usually available in emergency rooms for a half hour to two hours. During this time the doctor rapidly gives sodium chloride (salt) diluted in water into a vein (intravenous saline), and this nearly always increases the blood pressure to safe levels until blood is available. During the bleeding described, the kidneys also immediately start to retain sodium and water and return it to the blood; i.e., the kidney gives us an immediate transfusion of saline. Nature always finds a way of healing!

## Figure 13-2. Hypothesis for the Causation of Primary (Essential) Hypertension

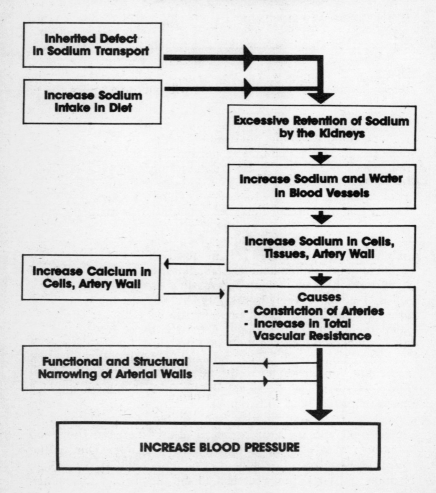

Increased salt intake is believed to be the most important factor causing hypertension in susceptible individuals. The evidence is strong enough to warrant general education of the public. The U.S. Food and Drug Administration, the World Health Organization, the American Heart Association, the American Medical Association, the National Heart, Lung and Blood Institute, and two government-sponsored bodies in the United Kingdom have advised the general population to reduce sodium consumption where possible.

There is a considerable amount of scientific information that supports the view that increased salt intake causes hypertension in susceptible individuals. I will outline a few of these:

1.  Population groups that consume very low amounts of sodium, less than two grams daily, have almost no primary hypertension; for example, groups in South America, Africa, and the South Pacific. In contrast, in countries such as Japan and Korea where sodium intake is excessively high, i.e., greater than six grams daily, hypertension is very common.
    The following evidence is cited by Dr. H. E. deWardener in *Lancet*, 1984.[1]

2.  Twenty-seven studies in human populations have shown a close correlation between sodium intake and blood pressure.

3.  There has been a fall in the incidence of hypertension in Japan between years 1971 and 1981, and this is believed to be due to a fall in the daily sodium consumption from above six grams to less than four grams.

4.  In Belgium between 1968 and 1981 a fall in daily sodium consumption from greater than six grams to less than four grams was associated with a significant fall in mortality due to stroke.

5.  In children of hypertensive parents, increased sodium intake causes an increase in blood pressure and a greater rise in blood pressure after stress.

6.  Compounds that cause sodium and water retention by the kidney (hydrocortisone, licorice) often increase blood pressure. In patients with Addison's Disease, low blood pressure is always present and is treated with cortisone. Cortisone retains sodium with water, and this

effect always increases blood pressure. Diuretic drugs cause the kidney to remove excess sodium from the blood and put the sodium and water out in the urine and thus cause a decrease in blood pressure.

7. Patients with chronic kidney failure who lose excessive sodium in the urine tend to have a normal blood pressure, but in those who retain excessive sodium, blood pressure is often elevated.

8. Animal experiments show a close relationship between salt intake and hypertension.

Despite the aforementioned points, incriminating an increased salt intake with hypertension, the Medical Research Council blood pressure unit in Glasgow headed by a panel of experts states that the evidence is unclear and unproven. Thus, they do not feel it justified to ask everyone to reduce sodium intake.[2] However, there is a consensus in North America and Europe that a moderate reduction in salt intake to less than two grams has no adverse health effects, and whenever possible, it would be prudent for the general population to reduce sodium intake, in particular, patients with primary hypertension and their relatives. If you have kidney disease, you should not reduce salt intake unless advised by a physician. (Some kidney patients can reduce intake.)

The evidence suggesting an inherited kidney defect stems from the work of Dr. Lewis Dahl, who bred two strains of rats, one that consistently developed hypertension when given an increased sodium diet, and the other that resisted the development of hypertension and never became hypertensive while on the same diet. Further, when a kidney is taken from a hypertensive rat and transplanted into a host rat with a blood pressure that is in the normal range (normotensive rat), the blood pressure of the host rat rises. A kidney transplanted from a normotensive rat lowers the blood pressure of a hypertensive host rat. It is believed that both the genetic and environmental factors (salt, stress, etc.) act together to cause hypertension.

Other hypotheses for the causation of primary hypertension are shown in Figure 13-3. Hereditary factors and stress cause an increase in discharge from a center in the brain (sympathetic center), which triggers the secretion of adrenaline and noradrenaline. These compounds cause not only an increase in heart rate and cardiac output, but a marked constriction of arteries and increased total vascular resistance, thereby increasing blood pressure. This sympathetic stimulation activates enzymes in the kidney and adrenal glands (the renin-angiotensin-aldosterone system) (Figure 13-3). Angiotensin is a powerful constrictor of arteries and thereby elevates blood pressure. Aldosterone, a hormone secreted by the adrenal glands, causes the kidney to retain sodium and water and this further increases blood pressure. However, the renin-angiotensin-aldosterone system appears to have only a small role, and this is still undefined in the causation of hypertension. A low intake of calcium has been associated with an increase in blood pressure in two studies, but the evidence is not sufficient to implicate a low calcium intake in the causation of hypertension. Further studies are necessary to clarify the aforementioned theories of causation.

## SYMPTOMS AND HARMFUL EFFECTS OF HYPERTENSION

Hypertension damages the arteries in many vital organs especially the brain, heart, kidneys, and eyes. Damage to the wall of arteries is due to the increase in blood pressure, but important added factors are an increase in pulsatile force and velocity of the blood. The artery wall responds to this stress by thickening its walls, but this leads to further narrowing of the arteries and a further increase in blood pressure. The arteries must branch to supply blood to various organs and tissues. Unfortunately, the branches to some areas take off at near right angles and mechanical stress is greatest at these points. The high velocity and pulsatile force of blood at a high pressure set up turbulence and mechanical stress that damage the smooth lining of the arteries, occasionally causing small tears (dissections) of the arteries. The mechanical injury provokes proliferation of smooth muscle cells of the artery walls and accumulation of fatty material including cholesterol and small blood particles (platelets). This thickening produces a plaque (atheroma) that juts out into the lumen of the artery thus obstructing blood flow, causing low flow and turbulence in the artery.

The term for hardening of the artery is sclerosis, hence the combination "atherosclerosis," meaning hardening of the arteries due to atheroma. This process is continuous over several years and produces no symptoms. However, on these plaques or damaged points, a blood clot (thrombosis) may eventually occur in vital organs such as the brain, heart, or kidney. In the brain a blockage (cerebral thrombosis) or rupture (hemorrhage) of an artery produces damage to a segment of cells, which results in weakness or paralysis of limbs and this is referred to as stroke. Each year about 500,000 Americans suffer a stroke, and more than 170,000 die as a result.

In the heart, the coronary arteries feed the heart muscle with blood. A blockage of a coronary artery by atheromatous plaque or clot causes damage to the heart muscle, and this is called a heart attack.

High blood pressure causes enlargement and thickening of the heart muscle. These changes may be observed occasionally on examining the patient or detected on chest X-ray or electrocardiogram. At some point in time, the heart muscle weakens and thus fails to eject sufficient blood into the arteries to satisfy the needs of the tissues, and this is termed a failing heart or heart failure. Blood that cannot be ejected into the aorta backs up into the lungs, causing stiffness of the lung tissue and leakage of fluid into the air sacs (alveoli). These changes in the lungs cause severe shortness of breath. Heart failure can be precipitated by mild hypertension in patients who already have a damaged heart muscle commonly due to an old heart attack (weakened scar). However, there are many other causes of a weakened heart muscle, and hypertension of all grades is detrimental in all types of heart disease. In blacks, heart failure is precipitated at a lesser degree of hypertension than in whites.

In the kidney, hardening of the arteries leads to reduced blood flow and chronic deterioration of the kidney function, and this causes a further increase in blood pressure. Fortunately, only in patients with severe hypertension is kidney failure a final occurrence. The vessels in the back of the eyes may be damaged by high blood pressure, and the changes may be observed by your doctor if he or she examines your eyes with an opthalmoscope.

Hypertension can weaken the wall of the aorta. The wall may balloon, and this is referred to as an aneurysm of the aorta.

The weak spot may rupture. Rupture is often catastrophic and the condition can be confused with a severe heart attack; fortunately, this condition is rare. The risk of narrowing or blockage of the arteries in the legs (peripheral vascular disease) is increased by hypertension, especially when there is either associated smoking, high cholesterol, or diabetes.

There is little doubt from the aforementioned points that hypertension either leads to early death or inflicts serious physical handicaps to millions. I am not a preacher, but I say: Save yourself. Blood pressure may be mildly or moderately elevated for several years without symptoms until the occurrence of stroke, heart attack, or heart failure.

*Symptoms* may not occur for five to twenty years in the majority of patients with mild and moderate primary hypertension. Headaches, dizziness, and nose bleeds occur with as equal frequency in hypertensives as in individuals with normal blood pressure. Only in a few patients can symptoms be correlated with the height of blood pressure. Because your blood pressure may be very high and yet produce no symptoms, it is necessary to have a blood pressure check once or twice a year.

## BLOOD TESTS AND OTHER INVESTIGATIONS

Your doctor will very likely ask you to have blood, urine, and other tests to determine if your hypertension is primary, i.e., without a cause, or secondary to diseases of organs, especially the kidney. The tests will also serve as a baseline for future comparison and as a means for detecting side effects of some antihypertensive drugs. The tests and the reasons for their use are as follows:

1. A complete blood count determines the number of red and white blood cells in your blood. The red blood cells contain hemoglobin; heme is the iron in your blood, and this is combined with a protein called globin. The level of hemoglobin will indicate if you are low in blood (anemia).

2. A test for electrolytes measures the amount of sodium, potassium, and chloride in the blood. The potassium

level in the blood is important as it may fall if you are taking a water pill (diuretic), which is commonly used to treat hypertension.

3.  Either the blood urea nitrogen (BUN) or serum creatinine must be obtained. Urea and creatinine are waste products excreted by the kidney into the urine. The level of these substances in the blood is fairly constant when the kidney is functioning normally, but rises in kidney dysfunction. Your doctor will be able to tell from the results of these tests, as well as from urine tests, if the kidney is the likely cause of your hypertension.

4.  A urine test (urinalysis) may show excess proteins, bacteria, or fragments of cells (casts) in the urine, indicating kidney disease.

5.  A chest X-ray is necessary and will tell the doctor if the heart is normal in size or already enlarged due to hypertension.

6.  An electrocardiogram can more accurately tell if the heart is enlarged and under strain. A chest X-ray cannot indicate whether the left ventricle of the heart is being strained by the high blood pressure. The ECG may also give other important information. The reassuring news is that other tests are necessary in only a few hypertensive patients, perhaps 5 out of 100 patients.

7.  Intravenous pyelogram (IVP). In a few hypertensive patients with suspected kidney disease, this test may be requested by the doctor. A dye that can be seen easily on X-ray is injected into a vein in the arm and reaches the kidney within a few minutes. X-rays of the kidneys are taken over a twenty-minute period. If the kidney is functioning normally, the dye is excreted into the urine and the X-ray will show the kidney structure as well as give some indication of kidney function.

8.  Special urine tests for the breakdown products of adrenaline (VMA, metaphrines) as indicated earlier are rarely required to exclude a tumor (pheochromocytoma) of the inner part of the adrenal gland, which secretes adrenaline.

A dye test showing the arteries of the kidney (arteriogram) may be required if your doctor suspects from the IVP that the artery to the kidney is obstructed. This is very rare, about 1 in 500 patients.

## TREATMENT CONTROVERSIES

The drug treatment of mild primary hypertension, i.e., a diastolic blood pressure recorded at 90 to 99 mm Hg in patients under the age of seventy, is a controversial subject. Many experts from the United States agree with the findings of the Hypertension Detection Follow-Up Program and recommend drug treatment based on the results of that study.[3] The implications for drug treatment made from the results of this study have been the subject of intense criticism.

During 1984 and 1985, many hypertensive specialists in the United States and the majority in Canada adopted a nondrug therapy program for the management of mild hypertension. Experts in the United Kingdom and elsewhere do not agree with the drug treatment of this group except in selected patients.

The cost of treating approximately 40 million mild hypertensives at $500 per patient per year is $20 billion per year. This is a considerable burden to both state and patient. Drug treatment of mild hypertension is unwarranted in view of inconclusive trial results. Drug treatment may be advised in mild hypertension in the following selected patients:

1. Patients who have had a heart attack, angina, enlargement of the heart, or heart failure.
2. Patients with an elevated blood cholesterol, for example greater than 265 milligrams per 100 milliliters of blood (mg/dL), with HDL ("good") cholesterol less than 35 mg/dL.
3. Patients with a strong family history of cardiovascular death or stroke before age sixty-five.
4. Patients in whom hypertension persists or has increased after one year of nondrug treatment. (The good news is that about 48 percent of mild hypertensives on nondrug treatment when reviewed at the end of one year are found to have normal blood pressures.[4])

If mild hypertension persists after one year or increases despite nondrug treatment regimens, I agree with the majority of experts who recommend drug treatment.

The British Medical Research Council Study on mild hypertension involving 18,000 patients and completed in 1985 showed that drug treatment of mild hypertension prevents the occurrence of strokes.

A diuretic (water pill) is the medication most commonly used as initial therapy in North America to treat mild to moderate hypertension. All antihypertensive drugs including diuretics carry potential side effects, making the rationale for their use in the mild hypertensive open to question—their use must be justified! Several studies, including the Multiple Risk Factor Intervention Trial (MRFIT), that involve the use of diuretics in hypertension show that these drugs may influence doctors to stop using diuretics as the initial therapy of hypertension, except in selected patients.

## NONDRUG TREATMENT

Since the majority of patients with mild primary hypertension are advised to persist with a one-year trial of nondrug treatment, it is important to understand the essential requirements of the program. The hypertensive must be aware of dangers of the so-called silent killer so as to become sufficiently motivated to comply with self-imposed treatment. Individuals who persist with nondrug treatment have a 50 percent chance of lowering blood pressure to normal. The essential requirements are given in order of importance, and each will be discussed in detail below.

1. Sodium in the diet must be reduced to less than two grams daily and at maximum three grams.
2. Weight reduction is absolutely necessary and is always associated with a fall in blood pressure.
3. Removal of stress or learning to adjust to stress may result in reduction of high blood pressure, and a trial of relaxation techniques can be useful in some individuals.
4. Regular exercise will assist with weight reduction and relaxation.
5. Alcohol intake should not exceed three ounces daily.
6. The patient should reduce coffee intake and must stop smoking.

## Sodium Restriction

Sodium added at the table is only a minor part of the daily sodium consumption. A teaspoon, 5,000 milligrams of salt (sodium chloride), contains 2,000 milligrams of sodium (i.e., 40 percent). The body requires an intake of at least 200 milligrams daily. The daily North American diet contains about 4,000 to 6,000 milligrams sodium (two to three teaspoons of salt). Clearly no one adds more than a teaspoon of salt daily at the table or in cooking for one individual. The remaining one to two teaspoons must come from the food we eat. The aim is to cut sodium intake by 50 percent, to two grams daily. This can be accomplished only if the hypertensive or potential hypertensive recognizes and reduces or discontinues foods that have a high sodium content. The list is long and contains many surprises (Table 13-1). The physician, the dietary adviser, and the patient must be alert, checking the sodium content of foods consumed during one-week periods. Foods that are not salty to taste may have a very high sodium content. Note that some puddings have more sodium than a helping of bacon. A large dill pickle has more than one gram of sodium. Fast food has a high sodium content (hamburgers one gram, three pieces of fried chicken two grams of sodium). Watch out for canned foods that have excess sodium added as preservatives.

Other high sodium foods not listed in the table include soy sauce, onion salt, celery salt, seasoned salt, salted crackers, pretzels, rye rolls, salted popcorn, most canned vegetables, sausage, hot dogs, salt pork, sardines, smoked fish, TV dinners, buttermilk, waffles, and pies.

It is obvious from Table 13-1 that the hypertensive individual must look at the food label and determine if it has a low or high sodium content. Anything that has more than 500 mg per can is high. Additives are listed on tins in order of greatest quantity. *Sodium benzoate, sodium nitrate, or monosodium glutamate means sodium*. Therefore, if any sodium compound is in the first five of the additives and the milligram content is not given, it is best to avoid the product. After a month or two of care, it will become second nature to purchase foods with a low sodium content. If you cannot avoid canned foods, rinse vegetables, tuna, and the like under running water.

Low sodium intake is possible if you use fresh poultry, fish, beef, fruits, and vegetables. Season foods with spices and herbs instead of salt and use a low-sodium meat tenderizer. Onions and raw tomatoes can be used liberally in cooking. All hypertensives should have dietary counseling at least twice yearly. The sodium content of several over-the-counter antacids, used for indigestion and stomach upsets, is high. There are, however, several brands on the market that have a very low sodium content, so please read the labels or ask your doctor.

Salt substitutes that contain potassium in place of sodium are helpful and can be used in place of table salt, except in patients who have kidney disease or take medications that retain potassium. You may need to try out several salt substitutes to find one that has a reasonable taste. Garlic powder but not garlic salt, onion powder but not onion salt, and chili powder may be useful to improve taste and yet remain low in sodium. Tomato juice and all the tomato sauces are high in sodium, but manufacturers are producing low-sodium tomato juices and a wide range of canned products.

## Weight Reduction

A loss of weight always produces a fall in blood pressure and is therefore strongly recommended. Weight reduction has a greater blood pressure-lowering effect than exercise or relaxation techniques and can be as effective as moderate sodium restriction. Dietary advice is given on page 78.

A weight-reducing, low-salt diet is often prescribed, but many patients fail to stick to a diet. Thus the diet must be individualized, and where physicians have little time to explain, it is best to refer to a dietary adviser, who can at least review the patient twice yearly.

Hypertension carries a greater risk of heart attack and stroke in patients with an elevated cholesterol. For patients under age fifty-five, the serum cholesterol should be maintained at less than 220 mg/dL. The risks are considerably increased if the serum cholesterol is greater than 260 mg/dL. It is important when following a weight reduction diet not to increase intake of foods that are high in cholesterol. Low-cholesterol diets and the optimal levels of total serum cholesterol and high density lipoprotein ("good") cholesterol are discussed in Part I. Weight reduction diets must be individualized; therefore, no specific recipes are given in this book.

## Stress

The role of stress in high blood pressure is difficult to define. What is important is the way we handle stress. Stress itself rarely produces sustained hypertension, but in a susceptible individual with an inherited predisposition to hypertension, stress may increase blood pressure (Figure 13-3). However, it is important to recognize that an individual with an average blood pressure of 135/85, when under stress, can increase blood pressure 20 to 40 mm systolic and 5 to 10 mm diastolic. These increases in blood pressure may last minutes or several hours several times daily, and play an important role over several years. Thus, the patient with mild primary hypertension on nondrug therapy will increase blood pressure significantly during the day under the influence of stress. The use of relaxation therapy has increased dramatically; many clinics offer facilities, although scientific studies have failed to show a sustained decrease in blood pressure due to therapy. On the other hand, studies are emerging that lend support to the salutary effect of relaxation therapy. Biofeedback-aided relaxation therapy seems to benefit some patients. This mode plus deep relaxation exercises are not harmful and can reduce blood pressure in some patients. Since the blood pressure tends to increase between periods of relaxation, do not rely solely on relaxation therapy if your blood pressure is greater than 160/100. Occasionally patients may need to change jobs or reduce workload, and to engage in hobbies, such as tennis, golf, swimming, fishing, painting, listening to music, or other forms of recreation.

## Figure 13-3. Other Hypotheses for the Causation of Primary Hypertension

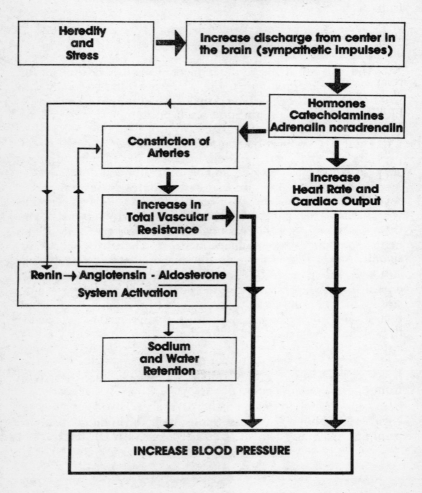

## Exercise

Isometric (static) exercise, such as weightlifting (pulling, pushing), increase muscular tension and constrict blood vessels, thus increasing blood pressure. Such exercises must be avoided. Isotonic or aerobic exercises may cause a variable increase in blood pressure during the exercise and slight decrease immediately following the exercise. Walking, jogging, swimming, and other forms of exercise should be encouraged in mild hypertensives. A fall in blood pressure may be related to weight loss and relaxation produced by exercise. If blood pressure remains elevated greater than 160/100 after six months of an exercise program, do not rely on exercise as a sole means to lower blood pressure.

## Alcohol

There is convincing scientific evidence that any more than three ounces of liquor daily significantly increases blood pressure. Therefore, alcohol should be restricted in all hypertensives. It is often stated that alcohol may produce relaxation, and two to four ounces daily may relax the nerves as well as increase the levels of HDL, the so-called good cholesterol. The risk of hypertension is greater than the possible benefits of a modest and variable increase in HDL cholesterol. If you have hypertension and previous heart failure, you should be restricted to the three-ounce limit daily. Five ounces of alcohol taken over a few hours cause a decrease in contraction of the heart muscle, thereby reducing the amount of blood ejected from the heart at each beat.

## Coffee and Smoking

Coffee is also known to stimulate the sympathetic nervous system and can cause mild elevation of blood pressure in susceptible individuals, especially if more than three cups per day are consumed. Tea has much less caffeine than coffee and is not known to increase blood pressure. Also, coffee increases blood cholesterol.

Smoking definitely increases the cardiovascular risk in patients with hypertension. Also, many drugs do not work efficiently to lower blood pressure because smoking interferes with their metabolism in the liver. The patient must therefore be motivated to discontinue smoking cigarettes.

## DRUG TREATMENT

### Which Drug to Choose

Your physician should strive to use only one drug in the treatment of hypertension whenever possible. The ideal choice is a drug that is effective for twenty-four hours when given once daily, and that produces little or no adverse effects. Several drugs are effective only for six to eight hours and must be given two or three times daily. This is more cumbersome, sometimes more expensive, and often results in the patient's forgetting to take the medication especially when the individual does not feel sick. Therefore, when possible, your doctor should choose a one-a-day drug for you. Occasionally the same drug is given twice daily and then once daily when the effective dose is achieved. However, this may not always be possible. A drug given twice or three times daily may eventually prove best for you; therefore you must give your doctor the opportunity to manage your drug treatment.

There are more than twenty-four antihypertensive agents. The doctor may state that the drug he or she is giving you is the best one for you. Yet on taking the drug, you may be the one to have side effects. Although side effects are fortunately uncommon and mild, you will need to discontinue the drug and try another. Thus, your doctor should explain to you some of the problems associated with drug therapy so that you will accept and comply with drug changes, which are often necessary.

The approach to drug management of hypertension in North

America is rapidly changing. The standard approach to antihypertensive treatment in the United States is to use a diuretic as the initial drug as dictated by a program called stepped-care treatment. This method has been in vogue since about 1968 and advises that a diuretic be used as the initial, "first-line" drug. If this fails to bring the blood pressure under control, then a "second-line" drug is added, usually a beta-blocker. If after several months the pressure is still not under control, a third drug is added, the choice being a vasodilator, to dilate the arteries. However, the stepped-care therapy is now under attack. In recent years beta-blockers have partially replaced diuretics as first line in Europe, and this change is slowly becoming established in North America.

Experts vacillate between one drug and another as to their choice of a first-line drug. Other drugs are now being tested for use as first-line. These include a new group of drugs called calcium antagonists, e.g., nifedipine capsules or sustained-release tablets that can be used twice daily. This drug is effective and safe for elderly patients and for patients with chest pain (angina), poor circulation in the legs, heart failure, or diabetes and where beta-blockers are contraindicated. Another important group of drugs that have proved beneficial in the treatment of moderate and severe hypertension are called converting enzyme inhibitors because they block the action of a series of enzymes (angiotensin, renin). Angiotensin causes powerful constriction of arteries and therefore increases blood pressure when the body requires a boost in blood pressure. By blocking angiotensin these drugs cause dilation of the arteries and a fall in blood pressure. In addition they do not stimulate the heart to beat faster as do some drugs. They also retain potassium while diuretics cause a loss of potassium. This group of drugs include captopril and enalapril.

The drug treatment of hypertension must be individualized. In order to assist your doctor to accomplish this goal, you must give your past history of illnesses and your response or bad reaction to drugs. In practice, a six-point checklist is helpful in the selection of an appropriate drug and it is useful for your physician to consider the following:

1. Your previous response or adverse effect to antihypertensive drugs should be a factor in determining further drug treatment.

2.   A beta-blocker (for example, propranolol or nadolol) is the drug of choice for you if you have angina or have had a heart attack or have a strong family history of heart disease. Patients younger than seventy years of age usually respond to beta-blockers; however, the blood pressure reduction appears to be less in blacks and in the elderly. Your doctor must respect the contraindications to the use of beta-blockers. In particular, he or she must not use beta-blockers if a patient has proven heart failure (a very weak heart muscle) or bronchial asthma. Relative contraindications include a very slow heart rate (less than 50 per minute), chronic bronchitis and emphysema, and very poor circulation in the arteries of the legs.

3.   If the patient has had previous proven heart failure, the doctor must avoid the use of beta-blockers or reserpine. Care should be taken with the use of hydralazine or clonidine. The drugs that are most suitable for this type of patient include a diuretic alone or combined with nifedipine, captopril or enalapril, and methyldopa.

4.   Patients with stroke or poor circulation to the brain associated with postural hypotension (a big fall in blood pressure on standing), should avoid the use of methyldopa, prazosin, or hydralazine and other drugs that cause considerable dilatation of the arteries on standing. Such drugs cause more blood to go down to the legs on standing and therefore steal blood from the brain, causing dizziness. It is important to note that beta-blockers do not cause postural hypotension and are therefore useful in this group.

5.   If you have very poor circulation in the legs due to blocked arteries, it is necessary to avoid beta-blockers, clonidine, and guanabenz. In this situation, I would strongly advise your doctor to use vasodilators such as nifedipine, captopril, enalapril, or prazosin.

6.   If you have liver disease, it is advisable not to take methyldopa, since this drug has been known to cause hepatitis, although this occurrence is rare.

Your doctor should arrive at a decision as to which drug to use after reviewing this six-point checklist.

Four main groups of drugs are in use:

1. Beta-blockers.
2. Diuretics.
3. Vasodilators (including calcium antagonists).
4. Drugs that act centrally in the brain.

Before we go on to briefly list the important drugs used in hypertension and some of their side effects and doses, it is wise to reflect on the following important question:

*Is the choice of drug or dosage really important in reducing blood pressure?*

Consider the following points:

1. It is not only the severity of hypertension that damages the arteries, but (a) the added pulsatile force of the blood; (b) the heart rate multiplied by the systolic blood pressure, which determines the workload of the heart and the amount of oxygen the heart muscle requires (thus an enlarged heart muscle working under strain will require more oxygen); and (c) the peak velocity of the blood multiplied by the heart rate,[6] which reflects the turbulence of blood (turbulence causes damage to the inner lining of arteries). These three parameters can be favorably influenced by beta-blockers, made worse by diuretics or vasodilators such as hydralazine and prazosin, and not altered by drugs that act centrally in the brain.

2. Beta-blockers are effective in preventing death in patients who have sustained a heart attack and are treated with these drugs for an additional two years.[7] However, only two drugs have been so studied in large clinical trials. Propranolol at a dose of 160 to 240 mg daily and timolol at a dose of 20 mg daily were effective. It is important for you to realize that we do not have any information regarding lower or higher doses. Consequently, the protective ("cardioprotective") dose should be used where possible in the hypertensive to try to prevent heart attacks or death.[8] The interest should be centered on the potential *complications*, and not just the blood pressure. The patient is not only

worried about his blood pressure but is afraid of stroke, heart attack, or death. Doctors sometimes lose sight of this goal.

3.   There is increasing evidence that diuretics increase cardiovascular "risk factors" and they may increase mortality.

a.   A fourteen-year follow-up of hypertensive patients treated with diuretics showed a major increase in the incidence of glucose intolerance, that is, mild chemical diabetes.[9] This effect was promptly reversed on discontinuation of the diuretic. Also, diuretics cause an increase in blood cholesterol and a decrease in HDL ("good") cholesterol. Thus, it is felt that diuretics lower the blood pressure, but could be increasing the incidence of cardiovascular disease.

b.   An increase in diuretic dosage will cause an increase in pulse rate, and this increases oxygen consumption by the heart muscle.

c.   Diuretics cause significant low blood potassium (hypokalemia), which significantly increases the irritability of the heart and may trigger off arhythmias and in rare cases death. The Multiple Risk Factor Intervention Trial indicates that diuretics may increase cardiovascular mortality.[5]

d.   The incidence of impotence is greater with diuretics than with beta-blockers.

e.   In a Veteran's Administration study, hydrochlorothiazide was shown to be more effective than a beta-blocker in the black hypertensive patient.[10] However, the latter needs further large-scale studies for definitive confirmation.

The answer to the question "Is the choice of drug or dosage important in reducing blood pressure?" is "yes." The available evidence suggests that beta-blockers have a definite advantage over diuretics as first-line therapy in a patient who is able to take either drug. When utilized, diuretics should be given in the smallest dosage necessary to control blood pressure; i.e., hydrochlorothiazide, 25 mg daily to a maximum of 50 mg. Hypokalemia (low serum potassium) must be avoided. A diuretic that conserves potassium such as Moduret or Dyazide has a definite place in therapy if you have normal kidney function (see "Moduretic," page 249, for contraindications to Moduret or Dyazide use).

## Beta-Blockers

See Tables 13-2 and 13-3 for dosage, and generic and trade names. Beta-blockers are excellent antihypertensive agents for the following reasons:

1. They do not cause a fall in blood pressure on standing unlike most other antihypertensive agents. (However, labetalol, which is really an alpha- and beta-blocker, does cause postural hypotension. This drug is useful in hypertensive emergencies.)
2. If there are no contraindications, the drugs produce no major side effects on the heart, liver, kidney, blood, or bone marrow.
3. A one-a-day schedule makes it less likely for the patient to forget to take the drug.
4. They can be used alone as first-line therapy in more than 60 percent of hypertensive patients under the age of seventy and used successfully in the majority of patients in combination with a small dose of a diuretic or with a vasodilator drug.

Commonly used beta-blockers include the following:

### Propranolol

This beta-blocker has been in use since 1964, and is well known to most physicians. The drug is metabolized in the liver. It is strongly fat-soluble and therefore has a high concentration in the brain. This may be the reason for occasional weakness and fatigue, the very rare occurrence of depression, and vivid dreams. Forty mg tablets are used twice daily and can be increased to eighty mg twice daily. Long-acting 80 or 160 milligram capsules are available for once daily use. Propranolol is the prototype of all the newer beta-blockers, and there are really only subtle differences. However, smoking decreases the effectiveness of the drug.

## Atenolol

Atenolol is totally excreted by the kidney and, because of a long half-life, it is given as a one-a-day tablet. It is different from propranolol and nadolol in that it is "cardioselective," i.e., affecting primarily the heart with only minimal effect on the lungs. Atenolol is therefore safer for patients with bronchitis provided that the dose is kept at a moderate level. However, if you have bronchitis it is best to avoid beta-blockers. Atenolol as well as long-acting propranolol and nadolol have been shown to effectively reduce ambulatory blood pressure for up to twenty-eight hours after the last dose. The effectiveness of atenolol does not appear to be modified by smoking.

## Metoprolol

Metoprolol is similar to atenolol in that it is also cardioselective at low doses. This drug is given twice daily. Other features of the drug are similar to propranolol.

## Nadolol

Nadolol is similar to propranolol except that it is not metabolized in the liver and is excreted by the kidney. Because of its long half-life in the body, it is given as a one-a-day tablet. Insomnia and vivid dreams occur much less frequently with nadolol and atenolol compared with propranolol and other fat-soluble beta-blockers, metoprolol and pindolol. Therefore, if you get bad dreams with propranolol, I recommend switching to nadolol, antenolol, or timolol. The drug's effectiveness does not appear to be affected by smoking.

## Oxprenolol

Oxprenolol is similar to propranolol but has mild stimulating properties, which is a disadvantage. A slow-release preparation is available for once-daily administration but may not last the full twenty-four hours. Oxprenolol taken once daily may not reduce blood pressure or heart rate during sleep.

## Pindolol

Pindolol carries no real advantage over propranolol and timolol. The drug may not decrease blood pressure or heart rate in hypertensives during sleep.[11] The drug causes significant insomnia, disordered sleep pattern, and in a few patients, nervousness, muscle cramps, and joint pains.[12]

## Timolol

Timolol has minor advantages over propranolol. The drug is six times more potent than propranolol, so for a given dose, a better blood level is achieved with less variation. The drug must be taken as 5 or 10 mg tablets twice daily. Because of its potency and lack of anesthetic property, timolol is used as eye drops for the treatment of glaucoma. Smoking does not appear to decrease the drug's effectiveness.

## Labetalol

Labetalol is a beta-blocker, but has an added action that causes the drug to block alpha-receptors. Thus, it is an alpha- and beta-blocker. It is useful in the management of hypertension of all grades, especially for hypertensive emergencies when it is used intravenously. The main disadvantages are that labetalol can cause significant postural hypotension and must be given two or three times daily in large doses. As well, the drug is relatively new and side effects may emerge.

## Advice and Adverse Effects of Beta-Blockers

Beta-blockers should not be taken if you have heart failure, bronchial asthma, or severe allergic rhinitis. Circulation to the skin may be reduced and susceptible individuals may develop cold fingers. This is not a reason to discontinue a very useful drug. Remember the saying, "Cold hands, warm heart." Therefore, if you are really distressed by symptoms that can be due to any drug, you must discuss this with your doctor so that he or she can select another drug. The drugs produce slowing of the heart rate, but this is a desired effect and a reduction to 50 beats per minute is acceptable. Rarely the pulse may drop to less than 45 per minute, and if accompanied by dizziness and low blood pressure, the drug should be discontinued. Fortunately, the latter effect is uncommon, judging from the millions of individuals who are taking beta-blockers. The drugs may rarely cause dizziness, occasionally weakness and fatigue, vivid dreams or insomnia, and very rarely mild depression. Reduction of libido and impotence are also fortunately rare. You must avoid stopping the drug suddenly because a worsening of angina can occur. This effect can be prevented by careful withdrawal over several weeks. This withdrawal phenomenon is important only if the patient has angina or severe heart disease and is not important in patients with hypertension alone.

Beta-blockers reduce blood pressure and slow the heart rate. Therefore, they reduce the work of the heart, preventing heart failure in virtually all hypertensives except the very few in whom heart failure has already occurred or the heart muscle is already severely weakened. A weak heart muscle may exist in patients who have had several heart attacks or who have severe heart valve problems. Such patients usually have low blood pressure because of the severity of heart disease. The aforementioned information, i.e., the patient's past history, makes it easy for the doctor to conclude that the heart muscle is weak, and this can be confirmed by the examination of the heart, the chest X-ray, and the ECG. It is important to emphasize that large clinical trials of hypertensives utilizing beta-blockers do not show an increased incidence of heart failure. Clinical trials with timolol, propranolol, and other beta-blockers in patients who have had heart attacks and were followed for two years showed that these drugs do not cause an increased incidence of heart failure. If patients are carefully selected by physicians, heart failure is not usually precipitated by beta-blockers and you therefore do not have to worry. This group of drugs is relatively safe and extremely important in the treatment of hypertension, angina, and heart attacks.

## Diuretics

There is no question about the efficacy of diuretics in mild to moderate hypertension, and when combined with other anti-hypertensive agents, they can be used in all types and degrees of hypertension. Thus, diuretics as first-line drugs in the stepped-care program have been regarded by many experts as representing a reasonable approach. The generic and trade names and maintenance dosage of diuretics are given in Table 13-4. They eliminate salt and water from the body via the kidneys and are commonly called "water pills."

### Hydrochlorothiazide

Hydrochlorothiazide is an example of a large group of commonly used diuretics called "thiazides," which I will not describe individually.
Supplied: Tablets: 25, 50, and 100 mg.
Dosage: Commence with 25 mg each morning and keep this dose as maintenance; maximum dose 50 mg daily, rarely 100 mg.
Action: The exact mechanism of action and antihypertensive effect is unknown, and the effect is believed to be related to:

1. A decrease in the blood volume. Patients who have an expansion of their blood volume especially due to sodium and water retention have the maximum benefit.
b. Increased excretion of sodium and water by the kidney.
c. Mild dilatation of arteries, thereby causing a decrease in total vascular resistance.

Contraindications:

    **a.**   Hypersensitivity to thiazides or sulfonamides.
    **b.**   Severe kidney failure.
    **c.**   Pregnant women and nursing mothers.
    **d.**   Patients taking lithium.

A decrease in blood potassium does occur in a significant number of patients receiving thiazide and this is a potential danger. Diuretics also cause attacks of gout. The drugs cause an increase in blood levels of uric acid, and urate crystals precipitate in joints, causing sudden severe pain commonly in the joint of the big toe or ankle. The joint becomes very hot, red, and swollen. Some individuals are very susceptible to small doses of diuretics and frequent attacks of gouty arthritis occur. Your doctor will prescribe a course of colchicine or indomethacin, and you will get relief in two to three days. Some doctors add to the diuretics a drug called allopurinol, and this is given for several years. It makes more sense to stop the diuretics except when they are required to treat severe heart failure. The addition of allopurinol is a prime example of "poly-pharmacy," which adds to the handfull of pills that patients are expected to take. It also adds to side effects and cost. I always advise patients to bring in "all" medications at each visit and these are reviewed. This verifies that the pharmacist released the drug prescribed. Drugs given by another specialist or the general practitioner may interact with the ones I prescribe. Drug interactions are a common cause of side effects that may elude physician and patient. I vividly recall the remarks of my professor in therapeutics (drug treatment), who made it a habit to remind us of the harmful effects of drugs. At least once weekly, his "good morning" to the junior staff on the patient's ward would be followed by, "What harm have you done today, Doctor?" His warnings have in some ways motivated me to write this book.

## Furosemide

Furosemide is a powerful diuretic and is not recommended for hypertension except when associated with kidney failure.

## Dyazide

Dyazide is a combination of 25 mg hydrochlorothiazide and 50 mg triamterene. The latter causes retention of potassium, and there is thus no need to take extra orange juice or foods with high potassium content. For dosage and side effects, see "Moduretic." Dosage is one to a maximum of two tablets or capsules daily. Larger doses should be avoided.

## Moduretic (Moduret in Canada)

Moduretic is a potassium-retaining drug and contains 50 mg hydrochlorothiazide and 5 mg of the potassium retainer amiloride. Dosage: One to a maximum of two tablets daily, although the manufacturer's dose is one to four tablets daily.

Dyazide and Moduretic are relatively safe when kidney function is normal; however, if kidney function is impaired such that the serum creatinine is greater than 1.3 mg/dL (115 umol/L), these drugs may retain too much potassium, leading to dangerous hyperkalemia (high blood potassium). The two drugs are widely used in the management of hypertension and heart failure, and prevent the patient from having to take unpleasant-tasting potassium chloride mixtures. However, diuretics such as Dyazide that contain triamterene should be avoided in patients who are being treated for arthritis with indomethacin, and should not be given to patients who have had a renal stone. Moduretic and Dyazide should be avoided if you are diabetic and over age seventy.

# Vasodilators

By definition vasodilators dilate arteries.

## Captopril

Supplied: Tablets: 25, 50, and 100 mg.
Dosage: 6.25 mg twice daily one hour before meals. If there is no major fall in blood pressure, the drug is increased to 12.5

mg three times daily to a maximum of 50 mg three times daily. However, a daily dose of 75 mg appears to be as effective as higher doses. It is advisable not to exceed 50 mg three times daily. If kidney failure is present, the drug is given only once or twice daily because it is excreted by the kidney and can be retained in excess in the body.

Action: As mentioned earlier, captopril blocks the formation of enzymes produced by the kidney and adrenal glands (see Figure 13-3). The enzyme angiotensin causes powerful constriction of arteries and increases blood pressure; when the enzyme is blocked, blood pressure falls.

## Advice and Adverse Effects

Captopril must not be taken along with potassium supplements or potassium sparing diuretics such as Moduretic or Dyazide since they cause a retention of potassium by the kidney. The drug may rarely cause a reduction in white blood cells, an increase in protein in the urine, loss of taste, and itching. A similar vasodilator drug, *enalapril*, with less side effects has recently become available.

## Hydralazine

Supplied: Tablets: 10, 25, 50 mg.
Dosage: 25 to 50 mg three times daily.

## Advice and Adverse Effects

This drug was used extensively from 1960 to 1966, but fell from popularity between 1968 and 1978, mainly because it produced significant side effects such as:

1. An arthritis-like illness (systemic lupus erythematosus).
2. Dizziness.
3. Postural hypotension.
4. Palpitations (tachycardia) and precipitation of angina in patients with coronary heart disease.

The drug is relatively ineffective when used alone, although it is effective when combined with a diuretic and is more effective when a beta-blocker is added in a triple combination. The drug is contraindicated in coronary heart disease, angina, and dissecting aneurysm. Many patients do not tolerate the side effects of hydralazine at doses greater than 200 mg daily and this dose should not be exceeded. Oral therapy, therefore, is recommended only when other regimens fail, and the drug is added at a dose of 100 mg daily to a maximum of 150 mg daily to a beta-blocker or reserpine, with a diuretic.

## Nifedipine (calcium antagonist)

This drug is a very useful antihypertensive agent and can be used for the management of all grades of hypertension.
Supplied: Capsules: 10 mg. Tablets: 20 mg (sustained release).
Dosage: 10 mg twice daily for one to two weeks; then 10 to 20 mg three times daily. I suggest a maximum of 80 mg daily.
Action: An increase in the amount of calcium in the artery wall causes a constriction of the artery and an increase in blood pressure. Nifedipine is a calcium antagonist; i.e., it prevents calcium from moving into the cells of the smooth muscle of the artery wall, thereby preventing contraction of the artery wall. The artery dilates and blood pressure falls. The drug can replace other vasodilators, such as hydralazine or prazosin, and can be used alone or in combination with a diuretic or a beta-blocker. The drug is of value in hypertension, especially in patients with coronary heart disease, in patients with decreased circulation in the legs, and when a beta-blocker is contraindicated.

### Advice and Adverse Effects

Nifedipine tablets twice daily as initial therapy have been shown to be effective in reducing the blood pressure during twenty-four hours of ambulatory monitoring. There are no absolute contraindications. The important side effects include headaches and dizziness in 5 percent of patients. The drug is a major advance in the treatment of hypertensives. It has no side effects related to the heart, lungs, kidneys, brain, blood, or bone marrow. In patients with severe hypertension, e.g., blood pressure 240/140, a major reduction in blood pressure is obtained by the patient biting a 5 or 10 mg capsule and holding it in the mouth for a few minutes. A reduction of from 40 to 60 mm Hg in the blood pressure may occur during the next ten to fifteen minutes.

## Prazosin

Supplied: Capsules: 0.5, 1, 2, and 5 mg (U.S.A.). Tablets scored: 1, 2, and 5 mg (U.K. and Canada).
Dosage: For mild hypertension, start with 0.5 mg test dose at bedtime. If there is no weak spell (syncope) or other adverse effects twelve hours later, then it is safe to take 0.5 to 1 mg twice daily for a week then progress to three times daily.
The average suggested maintenance dose is:

1. Mild hypertension—2 mg three times daily.
2. Moderate hypertension—5 mg three times daily (maximum of 20 mg daily).

A dose greater than 6 mg daily often causes an increase in heart rate and at this point the physician very often combines the drug with a beta-blocker, which decreases heart rate and further improves blood pressure control.

Prazosin blocks alpha-receptors in the walls of the arteries. Alpha-receptors in the artery wall, when stimulated, cause constriction of the artery. By blocking these receptors, prazosin causes the artery to dilate. The drug is thus a vasodilator.

## Advice and Adverse Effects

The drug has only minor side effects. However, an increase in heart rate is common, and while this may not be obvious to the patient, stimulation of the heart is perhaps not advisable. In this respect, the vasodilator drugs by expanding the arteries cause a fall in blood pressure similar to that of bleeding the patient. Thus this produces a reflex stimulation of the heart and an increase in heart rate. With hydralazine, palpitations may occur in 25 percent of patients, and with prazosin, 5 percent; however, more than 20 percent of patients with either drug will have an increase in heart rate.

## Drugs That Act Centrally in the Brain

### Clonidine

Supplied: Tablets: 0.1 and 0.2 mg.
Dosage: 0.1 mg at bedtime, and then increased to twice daily, with the larger dose at night. Maintenance dose 0.2 to 0.8 mg per day. The manufacturers have indicated a larger dose.
Action:
   Impulses or discharges originate in the brain (sympathetic impulses) and reach the arteries and cause them to constrict, therefore elevating blood pressure. Clonidine prevents the discharges or impulses from leaving the brain.

### Advice and Adverse Effects

   The drug is contraindicated in patients with depression. Drowsiness is increased by alcohol and tranquilizers. Dryness of the mouth occurs commonly, and although dry eyes are not common, the patient still requires periodic eye examinations when taking this drug. Also, a severe increase in blood pressure (rebound hypertension) can occur if the drug is discontinued suddenly. I rarely recommend this drug.

### Guanabenz

   This drug has similar effects to clonidine.
Supplied: Tablets: 4 and 8 mg.
Dosage: 4 mg at bedtime for one to seven days then 4 to 8 mg twice daily. A single bedtime dose is reported to be effective in some patients.

## Methyldopa

Supplied: Tablets: 125, 250, and 500 mg.
Dosage: 250 mg twice daily increasing over days or weeks to 250 mg three times daily; 500 mg twice or three times daily (maximum 2 g daily).
Action: It is postulated that the action of methyldopa is central in the brain, decreasing sympathetic impulse outflow.

### Advice and Adverse Effects

The drug should rarely, if ever, be used without diuretics because it causes significant sodium and water retention. The drug is a very effective antihypertensive agent when combined with a diuretic. However, because of the potential side effects, the drug is now reserved for treatment of moderate and severe hypertension when beta-blockers,[3] diuretics, or other drugs fail to achieve control. The drug has been used successfully for more than twenty-five years.

You should not take the drug if you have active liver disease or depression. The drug has been known to cause a mild hemolytic anemia, and so blood counts are necessary from time to time. If the drug is stopped suddenly, the blood pressure often increases over the next twelve hours to very high levels (rebound hypertension); therefore you must discontinue the drug gradually. If the dose is increased too rapidly, a sudden drop in blood pressure resulting in dizziness or a fainting spell may occur.

Other adverse effects include sedation and sexual dysfunction.

## Reserpine

Supplied: Tablets: 0.1 and 0.25 mg.
Dosage: Initially, 0.25 mg once daily for two weeks, then reduce to 0.1 mg daily for maintenance. Maximum maintenance: 0.25 mg with a diuretic.

## Advice and Adverse Effects

Contraindications include mental depression, active peptic ulcer, ulcerative colitis, and Parkinson's Disease. If the daily dose is kept at 0.1 mg or a maximum of 0.25 mg, the side effects will be rare. Depression occurs in approximately 10 percent with such doses; however, the drug must not be used if you have a history of depression. The drug has some advantages in that it is effective and economical and can be used once daily. The doctor does not have to increase the dose gradually over several months as is necessary with beta-blockers, prazosin, or most antihypertensive agents. Reserpine in combination with diuretics or hydralazine is available in a single tablet and is recommended when other medications are contraindicated or fail to achieve reasonable control, or are unavailable. However, the reserpine-diuretic tablets commercially available provide far too much of each drug when the dose exceeds one tablet daily. Reserpine has been rarely used in North America or Europe since the late 1960s because of the advent of safer alternatives. However, the drug is of value and rightly used in countries where high cost and/or availability of drugs pose serious problems for patients.

Other drugs available for the treatment of hypertension are derivatives of the ones mentioned above. I have limited the discussion to drugs that are useful and have a role in the treatment of hypertension during the 1980s.


## Conclusion

Mild to moderate hypertension should be treated with one of the following:

1.  Beta-blockers, especially for patients younger than sixty-five, and in all the patients with evidence of coronary heart disease or those considered at high risk for cardiovascular events (angina, heart attacks, cardiac death).
2.  Thiazide diuretics in small doses, with special care to avoid hypokalemia (low blood potassium). From 1966

to 1984, the usual dose of a diuretic, such as hydro-chlorothiazide, was 50 to 100 mg. This dose is now considered too large since it often causes a low blood potassium. The use of a diuretic as the first drug to be prescribed (first-line) is particularly suited for patients in whom beta-blockers are contraindicated, and perhaps in blacks since it has been shown in some studies that diuretics are more effective than beta-blockers in blacks. A combination of one plus two is used only when one drug has been adequately tried, keeping in mind the risk of side effects associated with the increased dosage of a single drug.

3. Other drugs are given a trial if beta-blockers and/or diuretics are contraindicated or produce adverse effects.

## HYPERTENSION IN PREGNANCY

The safety of antihypertensive drugs is always a question in the minds of a doctor and, in particular, the pregnant patient. There are only a few relatively safe drugs available for use in the pregnant hypertensive patient. Thiazide diuretics are contraindicated because they cause a reduction in blood flow through the placenta and can produce a decrease in blood platelets in the fetus. Many obstetricians are satisfied with the use of methyldopa or hydralazine, but beta-blockers, in particular atenolol, have had some favorable reports. If hypertension becomes severe during pregnancy, the patient is usually admitted to the hospital and most obstetricians give a trial of intravenous hydralazine.

## HYPERTENSION IN THE ELDERLY

Hypertension in the elderly (age over seventy) is established when three consecutive blood pressure readings exceed 160/95. Often the increased systolic blood pressure is due to the hardening and reduced elasticity of the artery and therefore requires more cuff pressure to occlude the brachial artery. In some elderly patients, the blood pressure taken by the cuff may give systolic values greater than 200 mm Hg yet intra-arterial blood pressure measurement often shows a normal pressure reading. This is called pseudohypertension and requires no treatment.

There are no scientific studies that show that drug treatment of the elderly patient with diastolic blood pressures less than 105 mm Hg significantly improves mortality in the elderly. No controlled, randomized trial has been completed for isolated systolic hypertension. However, there are reports of noncontrolled trials that suggest that treatment of moderate and severe systolic hypertension in the elderly does reduce the incidence of stroke and heart failure. A clinical trial is in progress in the United States. There is no formulated plan of treatment for the elderly; therefore treatment must be individualized. The following are suggested guidelines for managing hypertension in the elderly if the usual sodium restriction and weight reduction programs do not achieve a satisfactory level of control.

1. For diastolic greater than 110 mm Hg: Drug treatment is usually recommended.
2. For diastolic of 95 to 105 mm Hg: No drugs are usually given.
3. For isolated systolic hypertension with a normal diastolic, the systolic BP being 160 to 180 mm Hg: No drugs are recommended.

   For mild systolic hypertension, 180 to 200 mm Hg: Drug treatment is individualized.

   More severe systolic hypertension, 200 to 250 mm Hg: Drugs are usually required.

   For severe systolic hypertension, greater than 250 mm Hg: Drugs are usually required.
4. For a combined systolic of 180 mm Hg and diastolic of 110 or greater mm Hg: Drug treatment is indicated.

Many physicians elect not to treat mild systolic hypertension in the 180 to 200 mm Hg range in the elderly because there is no good scientific evidence to justify drug treatment. However, drug treatment is expected to produce beneficial effects in this group when the following conditions are present:

1. Heart failure, present or past, and/or enlargement of the heart.
2. Angina or past heart attack.
3. Previous stroke.

In blacks, the incidence of heart failure or stroke is much higher for a given increased systolic or diastolic blood pressure. Thus they may require earlier drug therapy.

You are strongly advised to take one drug only. If there are no contraindications, a one-a-day beta-blocker is worth trying although there is only a 33 percent chance of the drug's being effective in the elderly. If there are side effects, or there is a poor response in two to three months, the beta-blocker can be gradually discontinued. A diuretic that conserves potassium such as Moduretic may be tried if the kidney function is normal and you are not a diabetic. If kidney function is slightly abnormal, a plain thiazide at low dose is reasonable treatment. Too big a dose of diuretics would cause increased weakness, dizziness, and unsteadiness in the elderly. If you have angina, diabetes, or decreased blood circulation in the legs or have had heart failure, then 10 mg of nifedipine twice daily may be effective and safe to use with or without a diuretic. Many physicians have successfully treated mild to moderate hypertension in the elderly when it is necessary to do so, with one tablet of methyldopa at bedtime and a very small dose of diuretic, 25 mg of thiazide, in the morning.

Unacceptably high blood pressure should be reduced slowly without creating the risks associated with very low blood pressure. Thus in the elderly very small doses of antihypertensive drugs are used and only when necessary.

The treatment outline for the elderly is for individuals age seventy and over. However, most physicians agree that there is no reason to treat patients over seventy-five with drugs except in exceptional circumstances. Patients over the age of eighty are blessed with longevity, and doctors should not interfere with success.

## Table 13-1 LIST OF FOODS WITH COMPARATIVE SODIUM CONTENT

| FOOD | PORTION | SODIUM, MG |
|---|---|---|
| Bacon back | 1 slice | 500 |
| Bacon side (fried crisp) | 1 slice | 75 |
| Beef (lean, cooked) | 3 oz (90 g) | 60 |
| Bouillon | 1 cube | 900 |
| Garlic powder | 1 teaspoon | 2 |
| Garlic salt | 1 teaspoon (15 ml) | 2000 |
| Ham, cured | 3 oz (90 g) | 1000 |
| Ham, fresh cooked | 3 oz | 100 |
| Ketchup | 1 tablespoon | 150 |
| Meat tenderizer, regular | 1 teaspoon | 2000 |
| Meat tenderizer, low-sodium | 1 teaspoon | 2 |
| (Whole) milk pudding, instant | 1 cup (250 ml) | 1000 |
| Olive, green | 1 | 100 |
| Peanuts, dry-roasted | 1 cup | 1000 |
| Peanuts, dry-roasted, unsalted | 1 cup | 10 |
| Pickle, dill | Large (10 × 4½ cm) | 1900 |
| Wieners | 1 (50 g) | 500 |
| | | |
| CANNED FOODS | | |
| Carrots | 4 oz | 400 |
| [Carrots, raw] | 4 oz | 40 |
| Corn, whole kernel | 1 cup | 400 |
| [Corn, frozen] | 1 cup | 10 |
| Corned beef, cooked | 4 oz | 1000 |
| Crab | 3 oz | 900 |
| Peas, green | 1 cup | 5 |
| Shrimp | 3 oz | 2000 |
| Salmon, salt added | 3 oz | 500 |
| Salmon, no salt added | 3 oz | 50 |
| Soups (majority) | 1 cup (250 ml) | 1000 |
| Sauerkraut | 1 cup (250 ml) | 1800 |
| | | |
| SALAD DRESSING | | |
| Blue cheese | 15 ml | 160 |
| French, regular | 15 ml | 200 |
| Italian | 15 ml | 110 |
| Oil and vinegar | 15 ml | 1 |
| Thousand island | 15 ml | 90 |
| | | |
| FAST FOOD | | |
| Chopped steak | 1 portion | 1000 |
| Fish and chips | 1 portion | 1000 |
| Fried chicken | 3-piece dinner | 2000 |
| Hamburger | Double | 1000 |
| Roast beef sandwich | 1 | 1000 |
| Pizza | 1 medium | 1000 |

Table 13-2 GENERIC AND TRADE NAMES OF BETA-BLOCKERS

| GENERIC | PHARMACEUTICAL TRADE NAMES |
| --- | --- |
| Acebutolol | Sectral, Prent, Neptall |
| Alprenol | Aptin, Betaptin, Betacard |
| Atenolol | Tenormin |
| Labetalol | Trandate, Normodyne |
| Mepindolol | Corindolan, Betagon |
| Metoprolol | Lopressor, Betaloc, Seloken |
| Nadolol | Corgard, Solgol |
| Oxprenolol | Trasicor, Apsolox |
| Pindolol | Visken |
| Practolol | Eraldin (no longer in use) |
| Propranolol | Inderal, Angilol, Apsolol, Berkolol |
| Sotalol | Sotacor, Betacardone, Sotalex |
| Timolol | Blocadren, Betim, Temserin |

Table 13-3 DOSAGE OF COMMONLY USED BETA-BLOCKERS

| BETA-BLOCKER | DAILY STARTING DOSE, MG | MAINTENANCE DOSE, MG | MAXIMUM SUGGESTED DOSE, MG |
| --- | --- | --- | --- |
| Acebutolol | 100–400 | 600–1200 | 1200 |
| Alprenolol | 200 | 600 | 800 |
| Atenolol | 50 | 50–100 | 100 |
| Labetalol | 100–400 | 500–1000 | 2000 |
| Metoprolol | 50–100 | 100–300 | 400 |
| Nadolol | 40–80 | 80–160 | 200 |
| Oxprenolol | 60–120 | 120–320 | 480 |
| Pindolol | 7.5 | 10–15 | 15–30 |
| Propranolol | 60–120 | 80–320 | 320 |
| Sotalol | 80–160 | 160–480 | 600 |
| Timolol | 5–10 | 20–30 | 40 |

## Table 13-4 GENERIC AND TRADE NAMES OF DIURETICS

| GENERIC NAME | TRADE NAMES | TABLETS, MG | USUAL MAINTENANCE, MG DAILY |
|---|---|---|---|
| **Group I: Thiazides** | | | |
| Chlorothiazide | Diuril, Saluric | 250, 500 | 250–500 |
| Hydrochlorothiazide | HydroDiuril, Hydrosaluric, Esidrix, Esidrex Oretic, Direma | 25, 50, 100 | 25–50 |
| Bendrofluazide | Aprinox, Berkozide, Centyl, Neo-Naclex | 2.5, 5 | 2.5–5 |
| Bendoflumethiazide | Naturetin | 2.5, 5, 10 | 2.5–10 |
| Benzthiazide | Aquatag, Exna, Hydrex | 50 | 50–100 |
| Cyclothiazide | Anhydron | 2 | 2 |
| Hydroflumethiazide | Diucardin, Hydrenox, Saluron | 50 | 50 |
| Chlorthalidone | Hygroton | 25, 50, 100 | 50 |
| Methylclothiazide | Enduron, Aquatensin, Diutensen | 5 | 2.5–5 |
| Polythiazide | Renese, Nephril | 1, 2, 4 | 2–4 |
| Trichlormethiazide | Naqua, Metahydrin | 2, 4 | 2–4 |
| Cyclopenthiazide | Navidrex, Navidrix | 0.5 | 0.5–1 |
| Metolazone | Zaroxolyn, Metenix | 2.5, 5, 10 | 2.5–5 |
| Quinethazone | Aquamox, Hydromox | 50 | 50–100 |
| Indapamide | Natrilix, Lozol | 2.5 | 2.5 |
| **Group II: Loop diuretics** | | | |
| Furosemide, Frusemide | Lasix, Dryptal, Frusetic, Frusid | 20, 40, 80, 500 | 40–80 |
| Ethacrynic acid | Edecrin | 25, 50 | 50–150 |
| Bumetanide | Burinex, Bumex | 0.5, 1, 5 | 1–2 |

## Group III: Potassium-sparing diuretics

| | | | |
|---|---|---|---|
| Spironolactone | Aldactone | 25, 50 (UK), 100 | 50–100 |
| Triamterene | Dyrenium, Dytac | 50, 100 | 50–100 |
| Amiloride | Midamor | 5 | 5–10 |

## Group IV: combination I and III

| | |
|---|---|
| Thiazide and potassium-sparing | Aldactazide, Dyazide, Moduretic (Moduret) |

# CHAPTER 14

---

# HEART FAILURE

## DEFINITIONS AND CAUSES

Heart failure is usually the result of a diseased heart. The commonest cause is a very weak heart muscle. The heart muscle is the strongest muscle in the body. During an average lifespan, the heart beats about 2.5 billion times, pumping more than 227 million liters of blood. If this work could be accomplished in one moment, it would be sufficient to lift a weight of about 400 million pounds off the ground. If the heart muscle is severely weakened and unable to adequately expel the blood brought to the left or right ventricle, blood backs up in the veins that drain into the left or right side of the heart.

Oxygenated blood flows from the lungs through veins to the left atrium and left ventricle (Figure 14-1). These veins in the lungs can become overdistended with blood and leak fluid (sodium and water) into the lung tissue. This is termed lung edema due to left heart failure. If heart failure continues for several days, the fluid may also accumulate in the space between the lungs and the chest wall and this is commonly termed water on the lungs (pleural effusion).

The lung is like a sponge, and normally the spaces (air sacs, or alveoli) are dry and full of air. In heart failure, the excess fluid is in the spaces, as well as in the sponge work of the lungs. The lung is heavier; the fluid makes it stiffer with less capacity to distend with each breath; the individual therefore gets short of breath. The breathing is quicker and less deep

# Figure 14-1. Structure of the Heart

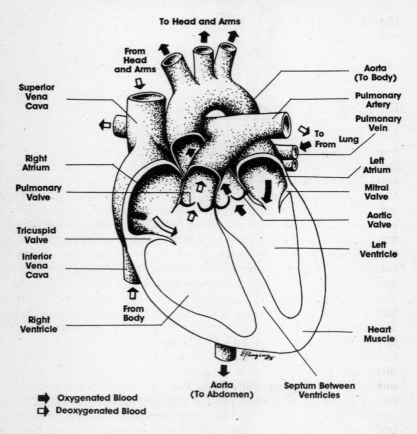

than normal breathing. The fluid in the air sacs and sponge work of the lungs consists of water, sodium, and some red blood cells. The patient may cough up sputum, which is sometimes blood-tinged. An individual with this type of condition is said to be in left heart failure or simply heart failure; because there is overdistension (congestion) of blood vessels and excess fluid in the sponge work of the lungs, the condition is also called congestive heart failure. I concur with doctors who drop the word "congestive," since heart failure can be present without congestion.

Heart failure is present when the heart is unable to eject enough blood from its chambers to satisfy the needs of the body. To reemphasize: In heart failure, blood and fluid overdistend or congest the veins that bring blood into the failing muscular chambers; this congestion or visible distension of veins is seen in the lung on a chest X-ray. In right heart failure, the distension and congestion occur in the veins of the neck, arms, liver, and legs. The examining doctor therefore frequently looks for these distended veins (jugular veins) at the side of the neck which take blood from the head and neck into the right side of the heart (Figure 14-1). When a normal individual stands, sits, or is propped up with the back and head elevated about 45 degrees, these neck veins are not visibly distended. In normal individuals they become distended temporarily when there is a marked increase in intrathoracic pressure as occurs during singing, trumpet playing, coughing spells, and the like. If these veins are distended and associated with shortness of breath, the doctor can be fairly certain that heart failure is present. What about nonvisible veins in the body? The distension backs up in veins within the liver, which enlarges, and in some cases, fluid may accumulate in the abdominal cavity (ascites). The veins of the legs may not be visibly distended but the blood is under back pressure and fluid leaks out into tissues, especially when the individual stands, walks, or sits for long periods. The swelling usually occurs more frequently at the end of the day, improves after a few hours in bed, and is best in the morning. The fluid around the ankles and feet is commonly called edema and is a hallmark of heart failure, although it can occur with obstruction of the veins from other causes. This fluid is similar to that described in the lungs, consisting of water and sodium; therefore, the legs are brine-logged not just water-logged. The swelling usually occurs in both legs whereas in obstruction of veins it is one-sided. The accumulation of several gallons of fluid may result in very extensive involvement of the entire legs, thighs, abdomen, and lungs. Edema was referred to in the past century as dropsy.

Left heart failure is most often due to extensive damage to the muscle of the left ventricle as occurs during one or more heart attacks. Patients recover within a few days as the muscle is able to function well enough in the majority. About 10 in every 100 cases of heart failure persist in a mild to moderate degree, and medications are necessary. With the occurrence of several heart attacks, some being silent, further damage to the muscle occurs, leading to very poor heart function and heart failure. Such patients should not feel that it is the end of the line; many can live for several years provided that there is adequate medical treatment. Surgery is not usually indicated unless the muscle balloons to form what is called an aneurysm. Fortunately, this is rare, occurring in about 1 in 10,000 patients with several heart attacks. If the aneurysm can be removed, a reasonable cure is possible with major surgery.

Heart muscle diseases (cardiomyopathy) not due to atherosclerosis of the coronary arteries or valvular disease are fortunately very rare. In rare cases cardiomyopathy can be caused by alcohol abuse. Viruses that cause a very mild or moderate flu-like illness can cause microscopic scars in the heart muscle and weaken the muscle sufficiently to cause heart failure.

The heart muscle is commonly weakened over several years by high blood pressure. The left ventricle has more work to do to pump millions of liters of blood against greater resistance through tight, constricted arteries. The additional work causes the muscle of the left ventricle to increase in size much like the increased biceps of a blacksmith or weightlifter. The heart enlargement (cardiomegaly) is easily seen on an X-ray. After several years, the muscle is strained, and the patient may suddenly be stricken by an episode of severe shortness of breath due to failure of the muscle and a back-up of fluid in the lungs. Incidentally, heart failure appears to be precipitated in blacks much more quickly than in whites at lower levels of blood pressure.

High blood pressure may be limited to the arteries in the lungs (pulmonary arteries) into which the blood from the right ventricle is ejected (Figure 14-1). Such a situation can occur in patients with severe emphysema in which many lung vessels are destroyed, thus increasing the resistance and blood pressure in the lung circulation. The right ventricle enlarges and finally fails, causing right heart failure.

Diseases of the heart valves, for example the aortic valve, can impede the free flow of blood from the left ventricle into the aorta; this is called aortic stenosis. When the mitral valve between the left atrium and left ventricle is tight, obstructing the flow of blood (mitral stenosis), blood backs up in the lungs and a cough with severe shortness of breath can occur. Other valvular diseases are discussed in Chapter 15. Other causes of heart failure are omitted since they are uncommon.

In addition to problems in the heart and high blood pressure, there are several factors, listed below, that precipitate heart failure when the muscle is severely weakened. *These conditions must be avoided or treated.*

## FACTORS KNOWN TO PRECIPITATE HEART FAILURE

1. Patient-physician problems:
a. Reduction or discontinuation of digoxin or diuretics. The doctor may reduce or discontinue digoxin or diuretics or the patient may stop taking the medications.
b. The patient may increase the intake of foods containing excess salt.
c. Increased physical exertion.
2. Increased cardiac work, imposed on the heart precipitated by:
a. A marked increase in blood pressure.
b. Abnormal heart rhythms; e.g., atrial fibrillation (see Chapter 15).
c. Pulmonary embolism (blood clot in the lung).
d. Infection; e.g., pneumonia, chest, urinary, or others.
e. Thyrotoxicosis (overactive thyroid).
3. Progression or complications of the basic underlying heart disease:
a. Acute heart attack or aneurysm formation.

b.  Valvular heart disease—causing increased stenosis or regurgitation.
4.  Drugs that weaken heart muscle contraction and may precipitate heart failure:
a.  Anti-arthritic (antiinflammatory) agents including indomethacin, ibuprofen, piroxicam, and phenylbutazone.
b.  Beta-blockers.
c.  Corticosteroids (cortisone, prednisone).
d.  Disopyramide (see Chapter 14).
e.  Calcium antagonists; verapamil and diltiazem.
f.  Stimulant drugs that increase blood pressure, e.g., adrenaline, amphetamine derivatives, and some cough and cold remedies.
g.  Alcohol, acute excess (e.g., eight ounces of gin in a period of less than two hours causes cardiac depression).

# MECHANISMS (PATHOPHYSIOLOGY) OF HEART FAILURE AND HOW THEY RELATE TO NONDRUG AND DRUG TREATMENT

When heart failure is caused by any of the diseases or precipitating factors outlined, the body defenses are called upon to assist. Nature always has counterploys. Heart failure causes less blood to be ejected from the ventricles. Instead of about five liters per minute being ejected at rest, the cardiac output can fall to less than two liters and not meet the needs of the body. Compensatory responses of the body are the following:

1.  The nervous system and adrenal glands are stimulated to produce adrenaline and noradrenaline. Adrenaline constricts arteries and, therefore, increases the resistance in the arteries, which increases blood pressure to allow survival. This increase in resistance is a great load, which can be likened to a steep hill, against which the left ventricle must pump. The muscle is already very weak, and the increased workload increases heart failure. Imagine a 1934 poorly tuned car trying to climb a long, steep hill. Nature's compensatory responses are

usually useful to the body, but in this case, they are counterproductive. The only way the heart muscle can do the work is to increase the contraction of the muscle and to reduce the resistance in the arteries. Nature unfortunately does not have a built-in answer and increases the resistance in arteries in order to increase blood pressure. The body is programmed to increase blood pressure when the cardiac output and blood pressure falls for any reason. Fortunately, medical scientists, by unraveling these mechanisms, were able to produce a series of drugs in the early 1980s that can reduce the resistance. These drugs are called vasodilators. Two important vasodilators, captopril and enalapril, will be discussed shortly.

2.  Two enzymes, renin and angiotensin, are activated. Angiotensin causes severe constriction of arteries and increases blood pressure. Renin stimulates the adrenal glands to secrete a hormone, aldosterone, which causes sodium and water to return to the blood vessels with the hope that blood supply and blood pressure will increase. However, the increased sodium and water returned to the blood by the kidney further increases leg and lung edema. Therefore, the body is once more deceived.

3.  The kidneys react immediately and utilize special mechanisms that cause a considerable amount of sodium and water to be returned to the blood vessels. The extra sodium and water again leak out of the blood vessels into the lungs and legs; thus, congestion and shortness of breath increases. You can understand therefore why doctors give diuretics, which cause the kidneys to excrete the excess salt and water and this relieves shortness of breath and leg swelling.

As mentioned earlier, adrenaline is secreted during heart failure and causes blood pressure to increase and the heart muscle to pump more forcefully. This compensatory response is helpful and in some cases bedrest and oxygen with this normal response may cause some relief. Drugs, such as Adrenalin, that increase the force of contraction of the heart muscle are called inotropic drugs. The best-known example of an inotropic drug is digitalis, which has been used for the past 200 years for the treatment of heart failure. You will note that the central cause is a low cardiac output, which seems to trigger the compensatory responses mentioned. Nature increases the blood pressure and heart rate but fails to increase the cardiac output adequately. It is blood pressure that is vital for existence. No blood pressure means no circulation to the brain and coronary arteries and, therefore, death. Researchers have endeavored to produce drugs that could increase the cardiac output when given orally without producing serious side effects.

## Digitalis (Digoxin)

In 1775, William Withering, a Birmingham physician, learned of a midwife whose herbal brew had cured several people suffering from severe swelling of the legs and shortness of breath. The condition at that time was called dropsy. Withering studied the brew and concluded that the only active constituent of the twenty or more herbs was derived from the foxglove plant (digitalis purpurea). He used the herb with a fair amount of success.

Digitalis has been used extensively across the world to treat millions of people with heart failure. The drug causes the heart muscle to contract more forcefully and increases the flow of blood to the kidneys. Congestion, shortness of breath, and edema improve. The drug also slows the heart rate and causes the heart muscle to use oxygen more efficiently. In some individuals, heart failure is precipitated by a very irregular heart rhythm called atrial fibrillation, and heart rate may increase to 120 to 200 beats per minute. In such patients, digitalis is very successful in reducing the heart rate to 60 to 90 per minute and causes complete clearing of heart failure. Digitalis remains the only available oral drug to treat heart failure caused by atrial fibrillation, and today this is its main indication.

Digitalis is not used in all cases of heart failure where the heart rhythm is normal, since in some of these, a diuretic suffices and in others the combination of a diuretic and a vasodilator "to level the hill" brings relief. A new inotropic drug called milrinone is now undergoing clinical trials in the United States.

The drug is about a hundred times more powerful than digoxin. In a study by Baim and others, all patients with severe heart failure not responsive to known methods of medical treatment showed improvement.[13] The drug causes an increase in cardiac output and relief of the symptoms of congestion such as shortness of breath and edema. Milrinone has very few side effects and has none of the serious adverse effects of digitalis. The discovery of milrinone is a major scientific breakthrough in the treatment of heart failure. The drug should be available for general use during 1987. Until milrinone becomes available, digitalis will remain the only approved oral inotropic drug.

Digitalis is available under various names. The most known and generally used preparation is digoxin.

Digoxin is the purest preparation of digitalis and gives reliable blood levels. Thus, I will confine most of the remarks to this preparation. Other preparations have very minor differences in absorption from the gut, blood levels, and duration of action. Digoxin is marketed under different brand names, in particular, the Lanoxin brand is commonly used in North America and in the United Kingdom.

Supplied: Tablets: 0.125 mg, 0.25 mg.
Dosage: For maintenance, 0.25 mg daily usually at bedtime. In patients over age seventy, 0.125 mg daily is usually sufficient.
Action: As outlined earlier, digoxin causes an increase in the force of contraction of the heart muscle and slows the heart rate, especially in patients who have atrial fibrillation. The drug is excreted virtually unchanged by the kidney. Therefore, in kidney dysfunction or failure, the drug accumulates and can reach toxic levels in the body. Patients with poor kidney function may therefore require 0.125 mg every other day or only twice weekly.

## Advice and Adverse Effects

Kidney dysfunction or failure is the commonest reason why toxicity occurs. Note that individuals over age seventy may have kidney blood tests (for creatinine) that are recorded as normal when the kidney function is abnormal. The doctor therefore has to titrate the dose carefully in the elderly.

Nausea and vomiting are common symptoms of excess digoxin in the blood. Blue-green-yellow vision may occur but reverts to normal as soon as the drug is stopped. Very slow heart rate, less than 48 per minute, with extra heartbeats and the precipitation of abnormal heart rhythms are common with toxic doses. If this occurs, the drug must be discontinued and levels in the blood measured. Low blood potassium increases all adverse effects and this may occur even with a small dose of digoxin. The potassium level in the blood should be checked every four months or more frequently in some cases. Diuretics are well known to cause potassium loss, and since they are virtually always used along with digoxin to treat heart failure, digoxin toxicity may occur, resulting in serious heart rhythm disturbances. Your physician will give advise on your diet, and tablets or a liquid containing potassium is required. Digoxin toxicity was common during the 1970s, and in the United Kingdom, where the drug was discovered, many physicians do not prescribe the drug for heart failure with normal heart rhythm because of the controversial benefit to this type of patient. In the United Kingdom, it was estimated that over 50 percent of elderly patients in nursing homes did not need the digoxin they were prescribed. However, several of these patients were really never in heart failure, and digoxin was used very loosely for the treatment of so-called heart failure in patients who had edema of the legs or some shortness of breath. I must emphasize that experts who have used this drug for over twenty years in patients with moderate to severe heart failure due to poor left ventricular function recognize clearly that when the drug is discontinued or the dose reduced, heart failure often recurs. I concur with this observation. Importantly, toxicity does not occur if the patient and a careful physician cooperate to prevent this.

## Digitoxin

Supplied: Tablets: 0.1, 0.15, and 0.2 mg.
Dosage: Initial and maintenance doses are the same: 0.05, 0.1 mg daily; maximum 0.15 mg daily.

Digitoxin has a prolonged action and the effects can last four to six days. It is broken down in the liver and excreted in the gut. Omission of a dose or kidney failure has little effect on serum levels. Levels are not usually increased in patients with severe liver dysfunction. The main "disadvantage" is that when digitoxin toxicity occurs, it can persist for several days.

## Capotopril and Enalapril

Captopril and enalapril are angiotensin-converting enzyme inhibitors and are useful in the management of all grades of heart failure. They are considered vasodilators.

Actions of captopril and enalpril:
As outlined earlier, in heart failure the body tries to maintain blood pressure at all cost in order to satisfy the needs of the brain and organs. The renin-angiotensin enzyme system is activated, since angiotensin is a very powerful constrictor of arteries and increases blood pressure. However, this increases the work of the heart and increases heart failure. Captopril and enalapril block a "converting enzyme" that converts angiotensin to its active component. This new group of vasodilators are therefore called converting-enzyme inhibitors. The drugs cause dilatation of arteries, reducing blood pressure and heart work. In addition, these drugs cause the kidney to return less sodium and water to the blood, further reducing the work of the heart. The drugs conserve potassium, and as mentioned, a normal potassium level is essential for the prevention of digitalis toxicity and the maintenance of the electrical stability of the heart.

### Captopril

Supplied: Tablets: 25, 50, and 100 mg.
Dosage: Withdraw diuretics and other antihypertensives for twelve hours, then give a test dose of 6.5 mg, then the same dose twice daily, increasing to 12.5 mg twice or three times daily, preferably one hour before meals.

The maximum suggested daily dose for heart failure is 75 to 100 mg. The 75 mg dose appears to be as effective as higher doses. The drug is excreted by the kidneys. If kidney failure is present, the dose interval is increased; for example, 25 mg three times daily can be reduced to 25 mg twice daily or to 12.5 mg twice daily. To reemphasize, in kidney failure less drug is needed at longer intervals.

### Advice and Adverse Effects

Captopril is not advisable in patients with severe anemia or severe renal failure. Do not combine with potassium in any form or with water pills that retain potassium. Severe itching of the skin and, rarely, loss of taste, increased protein in the urine, and reduction in white blood cells may occur. Blood tests are necessary from time to time to check the level of circulating white blood cells.

## Enalapril

Supplied: Tablets: 5 mg.
Dosage: 5 mg once or twice daily up to 20 mg daily.

Enalapril is a converting-enzyme inhibitor, and its effects are similar to those of captopril, as outlined above. However, the absence of a special sulfhydryl radical is believed to result in fewer adverse effects.

Other vasodilators used in the management of heart failure, mainly from 1978 to 1984, include hydralazine and prazosin, but their effects are variable and only rarely helpful. They are not converting-enzyme inhibitors and I do not recommend their use in heart failure.

## Nitrates

Oral nitrates, for example, isosorbide dinitrate, and preparations applied to the skin are described in Chapter 11. These preparations have a small role in patients who are not controlled with the use of digoxin and water pills, plus captopril or enalapril. Their main action is to dilate veins, pooling blood in the lower part of the body. Less blood returns to the heart, and congestion in the lungs may be slightly reduced. However, this effect is only a mild one, and the drugs lose effectiveness over a few weeks. They should be used in emergencies, in hospitals, or occasionally, at home to help patients with very severe heart failure get over a crisis. Try not to use the skin preparations for more than two weeks since they lose their effects.

Oral isosorbide dinitrate has a small role; the preparation is abused by doctors who add it routinely to digoxin and diuretics and even to the vasodilators mentioned. Patients may get weaker, feel dizzy, and faint. As well, the drugs cause severe headaches and add to the drug bill.

## WHAT TO EXPECT IN THE HOSPITAL AND ON DISCHARGE

The main symptom of heart failure is severe shortness of breath. Pain occurs only in those in whom heart failure is precipitated by a heart attack. If nitroglycerin is available, put one under the tongue and remain propped up in bed or sit until the ambulance arrives. Oxygen is most useful and is given immediately. Morphine allays anxiety and pools blood in the lower part of the body; both actions bring relief. Nitroglycerin paste, ointment, or patch is applied to the skin, and a powerful diuretic, furosemide, is given intravenously. Furosemide acts within minutes, pooling blood in the lower half of the body, and causes the kidneys to remove sodium and water from the blood and excrete them in the urine. Relief occurs within minutes, often before urine is passed. If relief is not obtained, further injections of furosemide are given.

The cause of heart failure and the precipitating factors are then treated, if possible; these details are beyond the scope of this book. Fast, irregular heartbeat, atrial fibrillation, is successfully treated with digoxin, as mentioned earlier. Hypertension can cause heart failure, and the blood pressure must be lowered. Preferably, captopril or a calcium antagonist, nifedipine, is used to dilate arteries, lower blood pressure, and thus rest the heart. Very rarely valvular obstructions occur, and when the patient is stabilized, surgery to open or replace the valve can be done. Patients with heart failure have a hospital stay of five to ten days. Prognosis depends on the cause and precipitating factors outlined. Heart failure does not mean the end. Some patients do much less than before but they can live five to fifteen years with good medical treatment. The reassuring news is that avoidance of precipitating factors can help enormously.

## ADVICE ON DRUGS, SALT, DIET, POTASSIUM, ALCOHOL, AND EXERCISE

1.  Medications must be continued as directed by your doctor. Do not stop any medications without consulting your doctor. Digoxin is usually necessary for a lifetime and diuretics for months to years and, in some, a small dose for a lifetime. I strongly advise you to take your medications with you on each visit to your doctor so that they can be rechecked or altered.

2.  As explained earlier, the individual must learn to live with a low-sodium diet. This does not mean that you must go to extremes and follow a diet sheet that outlines a 0.5 or 1 gm sodium diet.

    To achieve a low-salt intake, simply do the following:

    Do not add salt in cooking or at the table. If taste is a problem, use a salt substitute after testing several preparations on the market. Salt substitutes have potassium instead of sodium and are therefore better for you.

    However, if you have kidney trouble, you retain enough potassium; therefore, excess quantities are not required. The question of potassium and the kidney has been mentioned several times. I reemphasize that it is such an important and confusing area that both patient and physician must be careful. If you are taking captopril, enalapril, Aldactone, Aldactazide,

Dyazide, triamterene, or Moduretic (Moduret), do not use excessive amounts of salt substitute, eat a potassium-rich diet, or take potassium supplements without the advice of your doctor. Appropriate advice from your doctor depends on blood tests to evaluate kidney function and electrolytes, which include blood potassium.

Use foods containing small quantities of sodium. See Table 13-1 for foods with comparative sodium content. Low-sodium diets are discussed in Chapter 13, "Hypertension."

3. Apart from a low-sodium intake and an increased intake of potassium where necessary, the diet can be normal. There is no need to restrict cholesterol, fats, or sugars since this adds to the patient's misery for little return. Such strict diets may rob the patient of one beauty of life, that is, to be able to eat and enjoy a meal. This can result in a feeling of hopelessness and depression. Diabetics, however, still need to maintain their diets, but in heart failure, it is not necessary to be as strict because a higher blood sugar tends to cause a loss of salt and water from the body and this tends to relieve heart failure. There is no good evidence that trying to keep the blood sugar within the normal range or nearly so has any effect on survival, especially in the group of individuals with heart failure. Patients must lose excess weight to decrease the work of a failing heart. Less weight always causes less shortness of breath.

4. As outlined earlier, the level of potassium in the blood must be kept within the upper normal range, 4 to 5 mEq/L. Except when kidney failure is present, extra potassium is often required in liquid or tablet form. The tablets or capsules may cause some gastrointestinal irritation. In addition, the pills are large in size and often rejected by patients, and they contain very little potassium. When a patient has a low blood potassium and kidney failure is absent, I strongly advise a potassium-rich diet because the liquid medications have such an unpleasant taste. Foods containing a liberal amount of potassium are given in Table 14-1.

The intake of foods listed can prevent the use of

potassium pills or liquids. As an alternative, many doctors, including myself, advise a diuretic that retains potassium such as Moduretic or Dyazide. In moderate to severe heart failure, a combination of furosemide, which causes a loss of potassium, and captopril or enalapril, which retains potassium, is advised. The various diuretics are discussed in Chapter 13 in the treatment of hypertension. Potassium chloride mixtures and tablets are given in Table 14-2. To be useful, the preparation must contain sufficient potassium with chloride.

5. Alcohol causes the heart muscle to pump less forcefully. Eight ounces of gin given to normal healthy students caused a 33 percent reduction in the amount of blood ejected from the heart. Can you imagine a sick heart with a handicap? If you have had heart failure, either do not drink alcohol at all or keep it under two ounces of alcohol, a pint of beer, or four ounces of wine, two or three times weekly. Patients who have alcoholic heart muscle disease (alcoholic cardiomyopathy) should never drink alcohol.

6. Exercise or unaccustomed activity imposes increased work on a weak heart muscle and often precipitates heart failure. Walking is the safest and best exercise. Try to walk a half to one mile and stop and rest if you get short of breath. I do not recommend longer walks of two to five miles or jogging for patients with heart failure. Stooping and bending exercises may cause some dizziness especially if you are on vasodilators, diuretics, and nitrates. Patients with heart failure, especially if recurrent, are not advised to engage in exercise programs even if they are claimed to be rehabilitation programs. You can only strain the heart muscle; you could never improve it. I must reemphasize that the heart failure that occurs during an acute heart attack is completely different and often clears within one week. Such patients can engage in various exercise programs discussed in Chapter 10.

## CONCLUSION

Patients with heart failure can take hope since modern scientific discoveries have produced new types of drugs. Vasodilators, in the form of captopril and enalapril, have proved to be most useful in clearing heart failure and allowing patients to enjoy a fuller life.

### Table 14-1 POTASSIUM-RICH FOODS

| | | |
|---|---|---|
| Orange juice | Half cup | 6 mEq |
| Milk (skim-powdered) | Half cup | 27 mEq |
| Milk (whole-powdered) | Half cup | 20 mEq |
| Melon (honeydew) | Quarter | 13 mEq |
| Banana | One | 10 mEq |
| Tomato | One | 6 mEq |
| Celery | One | 5 mEq |
| Spinach | Half cup | 8 mEq |
| Potato (baked) | Half | 13 mEq |
| Beans | Half cup | 10 mEq |
| Strawberries | Half cup | 3 mEq |

Avocado, meats, and shellfish are rich in potassium.

## Table 14-2 POTASSIUM SUPPLEMENTS

| Liquids | Ingredients | K+ mEq (mmol) | Cl– mEq (mmol) |
|---|---|---|---|
| Kay Ciel; Kay-Cee-L 1 mmol/L | KCl | 20 | 20 |
| Potassium chloride 10% | KCl | 20 | 20 |
| K-Lor (paquettes) | KCl | 20 | 20 |
| K-Lyte Cl | KCl | 25 | 25 |
| Kaochlor 10% (or sugar free) | KCl | 20 | 20 |
| Klorvess 10% | KCl | 20 | 20 |
| Kolyum | KCl | 20 | 3* |
| Kaon Elixir | K gluconate | 20 | —* |
| Kaon-Cl 20% | KCl | 40 | 40 |
| K-Lyte (effervescent) | $KH_2CO_3$ | 25 | —* |
| Potassium Triplex | not KCl | 15 | —* |
| Potassium Sandoz | KCl | 12 | 8* |
| Rum K | KCl | 20 | 20 |

### TABLETS/CAPSULES—SLOW RELEASE

| | | | |
|---|---|---|---|
| K-Long | KCl | 6* | 6 |
| Kalium durules | KCl | 10* | 10 |
| Kaon | K gluconate | 5* | — |
| Leo K | KCl | 8 | 8* |
| Micro K | KCl | 8* | 8 |
| Nu-K | K | 8 | 8* |
| Sando K | K | 12 | 8* |
| Slow-K | KCl | 8* | 8* |

*Note the low potassium and/or chloride content of some preparations.
Dosage: Usual range 20–60 mEq (mmol) potassium daily.
K+ = potassium.
Cl = chloride.

# CHAPTER 15

---

# ABNORMAL HEART RHYTHMS—PALPITATIONS

The sinus node, a very small group of specialized cells, is located in the upper right corner of the heart (Figure 15-1). The node is about thirty millimeters long by three millimeters thick. Through its genetic code and the influx and efflux of sodium and potassium into its cells, this natural pacemaker spontaneously fires electrical discharges that are conducted through electric cable-like bundles to the atria and ventricles and causes the heart muscle to contract about seventy times a minute. The rate slows or gets faster depending on the needs of the body. The sinus node is like a powerful generator and has complete control of the heart rate. Cells outside the sinus node pacemaker, for example, ventricular muscle cells, possess pacemaker activity that is so weak that the normal electrical discharge from the sinus node suppresses them.

Occasionally, the sinus node is diseased and stops working for a few seconds and pacemaker cells that are normally suppressed give off escaped beats. These pacemaker cells may interrupt the normal heartbeat causing an extra beat (see Figure 15-1).

The electrical conducting system of the heart is vital to life. Damage to the electrical system can occur when the coronary arteries are blocked and fail to supply sufficient blood to the electrical system as may happen after several heart attacks. The electrical system can also be affected by certain degenerative diseases that cause calcification and hardening (sclerosis) of the bundles, and this may interrupt the electrical discharge.

281

# Figure 15-1 Electrical System of the Heart

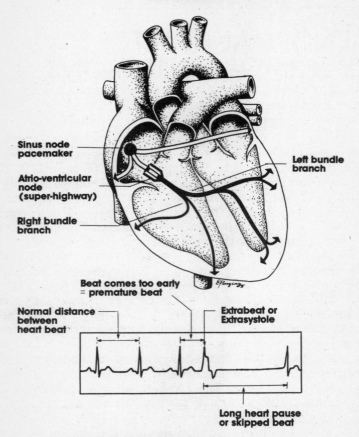

Sinus node pacemaker

Atrio-ventricular node (super-highway)

Right bundle branch

Left bundle branch

Beat comes too early = premature beat

Normal distance between heart beat

Extrabeat or Extrasystole

Long heart pause or skipped beat

The Electrocardiogram picks up the heart's electrical impulses transmitted through the skin of the chest. Premature beat is synonymous with terms Extra beat, extrasystole, heart pause or skipped beats.

# PALPITATIONS—EXTRA BEATS, IRREGULAR BEATS

The word "palpitation" is used by doctors and by some patients to describe the heartbeat when it is fast, pounding, skipping, or irregular. A patient posed the following question: I am twenty-eight and have a problem with a heartbeat pause. This problem comes and goes and may result in five to ten pauses each minute. Sometimes my heart feels as if it makes an extra beat. If I lie down, the irregularity seems more pronounced. I went to my family doctor, who found nothing wrong. My doctor concluded that these pauses were caused by too much adrenaline in the blood. Could you tell me more about this, the possible causes, cures, and long-term harm to the heart? I answered this question as follows: A heartbeat pause is due to an extra beat (extrasystole), medically termed a premature beat (Figure 15-1). Premature beats generally originate in the top chamber of the heart. These are referred to as atrial premature beats and they are of no significance if they occur in a normal heart. If they occur in a lower chamber, they are called ventricular premature beats. Patients perceive the abnormal heart rhythm as either an extra beat or a pause. An individual may state, "My heart skipped a beat." The extra heartbeat nearly always becomes more prominent when the heart slows while sitting or lying. When the heart speeds up during walking or other activities, the extra beats are suppressed by the normal beats. Movement of the body also prevents the sensation of the stronger heartbeat.

Premature beats may be due to either heart disease or extracardiac conditions, but often, they have no definable cause. Heart diseases that affect the heartbeat include disturbance of the blood supply to the heart due to coronary heart disease; diseases of the heart valves, usually due to prior rheumatic fever, or a common condition called mitral valve prolapse syndrome. Valve problems are easily excluded by a physician, who can hear murmurs or clicks when listening with the stethoscope. Echocardiography (cardiac ultrasound) can clarify the cause. Heart muscle diseases (cardiomyopathy) are fortunately rare. Alcohol abuse can, now and then, cause a cardiomyopathy. Viruses that cause a flu-like illness can produce microscopic scars in the heart muscle (myocarditis) that may trigger off extra beats. Myocarditis can be difficult to exclude if the patient is not seen during the acute phase.

Investigations of the patient with extra beats should include blood tests (to exclude anemia, a low serum potassium, or thyroid overactivity), chest X-ray, echocardiography, Holter monitor (24-hour ECG recording), and a stress test.

Extracardiac conditions include alcohol abuse, smoking, stimulants such as caffeine, amphetamines (diet pills), and nicotinic acid in megavitamins. In susceptible individuals, disturbances of the heartbeat (arrhythmias) are more common twelve to twenty-four hours after alcohol consumption. Other causes include low oxygen in the blood due to lung diseases and thyroid overactivity.

Extra beats commonly occur in young individuals with normal hearts and cause no harmful effects. In the normal heart, they bear no relation to heart attacks, sudden cardiac death, or heart failure, and they do not produce harm to the heart.

Drug treatment is not indicated for patients with a normal heart since the side effects outweigh the benefits. Some patients, who are terribly bothered by numerous extra beats in the presence of a normal heart or mitral valve prolapse, respond to beta-blockers. The presence of five to fifteen pauses per minute in a normal heart is of no significance and requires no drug treatment.

Patients may have an extra beat that occurs after each normal heartbeat and more commonly after two normal beats. Those who have episodes of very fast heartbeat, usually 150 to 180 beats per minute, may have a condition known as paroxysmal atrial tachycardia. If episodes are frequent, drug treatment may be necessary. The condition is discussed later in the chapter.

There is no conclusive evidence that excessive adrenaline triggers paroxysmal atrial tachycardia or extra beats. In a few individuals, excessive adrenaline may play a role during stress or during a heart attack. Beta-blockers can be useful when stress or heart attack precipitates extra beats. Excessive adrenaline is liberated in the heart muscle during a heart attack and does increase the occurrence of extra beats and other abnormal heart rhythms.

In the majority of individuals with extra beats, there is no good reason why they should occur at a particular time of the day or month. I explain to my patients that it is like having an itchy spot in the elbow crease that can come and go a few times per month or year. A microscopic area in the heart has an "itchy spot." I have never heard of an itch that killed anyone! Several studies have utilized the twenty-four-hour Holter monitor to show that more than 66 percent of normal individuals studied have extra beats arising from the ventricles (ventricular premature beats). I emphasize, that unless serious heart disease is present, all the bumpings, flutterings, thumpings, and irregular beats can be ignored.

# WHAT IS TACHYCARDIA?

This is the term used by the medical profession to describe a fast heart rate, greater than 100 per minute, with the individual at rest. I will describe five types of tachycardia:

1. Sinus tachycardia.
2. Paroxysmal atrial tachycardia (PAT).
3. Atrial fibrillation.
4. Wolff-Parkinson-White Syndrome.
5. Ventricular tachycardia.

## Sinus Tachycardia

When the fast beat arises from the sinus node pacemaker, it is called a sinus tachycardia, which is a normal occurrence during exercise and infections causing fever and the like.

## Paroxysmal Atrial Tachycardia (PAT)

This is one of the commonest abnormal tachycardias occurring in young healthy adults. Pacemaker cells outside the sinus node commence an electrical discharge and take over the heart rhythm for a few minutes to a few hours. One of my patients, Mrs. MH, age sixty-six, can recall having PAT from age twenty-two. Without warning, she would feel a sudden pounding of the heart. The beats were so rapid that it was difficult to count them. She would try certain maneuvers such as lying down, walking around, or taking a warm drink, all to no avail. Attacks would come on once or twice a year; in one year she had five episodes; the duration of the attacks was usually from several minutes to three or four hours.

She was age thirty-eight when she presented herself at the emergency room because the particular episode had gone on for more than three hours. The episode stopped a few minutes after she came to the emergency room. She was informed that she had PAT. Her attacks have a typical sudden onset with a rapid heart rate and abrupt cessation. Occasionally she feels dizzy, as if she is about to faint, but she has never really lost consciousness. I saw MH in the emergency room during one of her attacks. I reassured her that PAT nearly always occurs in a normal heart and this was the situation in her case. In addition, in a normal heart, PAT does not cause heart failure or angina, nor does it lead to a heart attack. She was at that time being treated with quinidine and had nausea and diarrhea. We advised her how she might suppress the attacks through the use of certain maneuvers that increase the activity of the vagus nerve. The vagus nerve is like the reins of a horse; it slows the heart and keeps it in check.

Simple maneuvers to suppress PAT are:

1. Gagging: Putting a finger at the back of the tongue to produce retching.
2. Holding both nostrils tightly and breathing out against the resistance for about thirty seconds.
3. Holding the breath and emersing the face in cold water for about ten seconds.

She was warned not to apply pressure on the eyeball. This was used by some several years ago, but it is not recommended since detachment of the retina may occur.

On a few occasions we were able to stop her attacks in the emergency room by massaging her right carotid artery in the neck (carotid sinus) for three to six seconds. This stimulates the vagus nerve and suddenly stops the abnormal fast heart rhythm in more than 50 percent of individuals. However, the technique should not be tried until the patient is hooked up to a cardiac monitor or electrocardiogram. If these facilities are not available, someone needs to listen to the heartbeat while the doctor presses the carotid sinus. The technique is not used in individuals over age sixty or in those whose carotid arteries are known to have obstruction by atheroma.

Mrs. MH's attacks became more frequent after age fifty, and I tried her on digoxin, which was a 75 percent success for one to two years. She later required a beta-blocker, which often helps this situation. You will recall that beta-blockers slow the heart rate. Very rarely a combination of digoxin and beta-blocker is necessary to suppress attacks, and this was tried with success for one to two years. Finally, she was tried on a beta-blocker alone and this was sufficient, except for two or three episodes per year when she would go to the emergency room; attacks would subside fairly quickly with treatment given.

The majority of patients with PAT get immediate relief in the emergency room when given a calcium antagonist, verapamil, intravenously. However, the drug cannot be used intravenously in individuals who have heart failure or who have a weak heart muscle, because it can precipitate heart failure in such cases. The drug should not be used intravenously in patients maintained on beta-blockers and those who are suspected to have digoxin toxicity.

## Atrial Fibrillation

This is a very common abnormal heart rhythm, which is completely irregular. The condition usually occurs after age thirty and can be due to previous rheumatic fever that damaged the valve and left scars in the atria. The atrium beats extremely fast, about 400 to 600 times per minute; however, the impulses that arise from these beats, occurring outside the sinus node, cannot all pass through the atrioventricular node. The atrioventricular node is like a superhighway that leads to the ventricle (Figure 15-1). At most, it can manage to carry 200 to 220 cars. Therefore, 400 or more cars cause a traffic jam, and in an erratic fashion, only a few can reach the ventricle. The ventricles therefore beat at 100 to 200 per minute, but very irregularly. The condition is usually treated with digoxin, which causes a block in the superhighway (atrioventricular node) and allows less traffic to reach the ventricles. Therefore instead of the ventricles beating at 100 to 200 per minute, it beats at 60 to 100 per minute.

Atrial fibrillation can on rare occasions occur during a heart attack and in other conditions such as an overactive thyroid (thyrotoxicosis) and occasionally in severe lung diseases when there is chronic oxygen lack. The condition is usually kept under control and patient's activities are not curtailed. If there is no serious underlying heart disease, lifespan can be normal. The condition is not to be confused with the dangerous ventricular fibrillation.

## Wolff-Parkinson-White Syndrome (DPW)

This is a form of tachycardia that is similar to PAT and occurs extremely rarely. In this condition, there is an extra electrical bundle running from the atrium to the ventricle. Conduction of impulses occurs much more quickly through this accessory or anomolous bundle, whereas the atrioventricular node tends to impede traffic and so maintain a slow heart rate. This condition has a typical ECG appearance and the heart rate maybe as fast as 200 to 250 per minute. Special drugs are now available to treat this abnormal rhythm, and in rare cases, the accessory bundle may have to be divided surgically.

## Ventricular Tachycardia

By definition, more than three extra ventricular beats occurring together constitutes ventricular tachycardia. This is a serious abnormal heart rhythm and occurs mainly in patients with severe coronary artery disease or severe disease of the heart muscle. The heartbeat is regular but fast, between 120 and 200 per minute, and usually the diagnosis is easily known from the ECG appearance. During a heart attack, ventricular tachycardia may occur and it is usually treated with a drug called lidocaine, followed by other drugs to suppress this rhythm. If success is not obtained, the patient's abnormal heart rhythm is converted to normal sinus rhythm with the use of a cardioverter, which delivers small electrical shocks to the heart. Such a cardioversion is carried out in the emergency room or the coronary care unit after the patient has had sedation with valium or another similar sedative. The patient therefore feels no pain.

*Two common conditions that are due to electrical distur-bances in the heart but unrelated to tachycardia or heart rate include:*

## 1. Right Bundle Branch Block (RBBB)

This is an ECG diagnosis. The electrical bundles which take the electrical impulses to the right ventricle are damaged and the electrical impulses fail to reach the right ventricle. The condition is not uncommon and can be seen in normal patients. However, it is most often seen with coronary heart disease, valvular heart disease, and lung disease. The heart rate re-mains normal.

## 2. Left Bundle Branch Block (LBBB)

This condition is not uncommon and similarly is due to a block of the conduction in the bundle that receives impulses from the atrium across the left ventricle. The ECG is typical and the doctor makes the diagnosis only after looking at the electrocardiogram. Right bundle branch block is often seen in normal individuals. Left bundle branch block, on the other hand is more often due to subtle diseases of the heart including coronary heart disease, valvular heart disease, and muscle scars. Left or right bundle branch block does not cause any distur-bance in the heart rate and does not require an artificial pacemaker.

# DRUGS TO TREAT ABNORMAL HEART RHYTHMS

## Digoxin

Digoxin is used to treat patients with recurrent attacks of paroxysmal atrial tachycardia as described earlier. The drug is used daily for a prolonged period, and recurrent attacks are prevented in more than 75 percent of individuals. The important role of digoxin in slowing the heart rate in patients with atrial fibrillation with or without heart failure has been discussed earlier.

## Beta-Blockers

Beta-blockers are occasionally used to treat PAT and are successful in more than 60% of cases. As well, the drugs can be used to treat bothersome extra beats (ventricular premature beats) when they are associated with increased secretion of adrenaline and in individuals who have a minor defect of the mitral valve, termed mitral valve prolapse. The drug has a beneficial effect on extra beats produced during a heart attack or when they are associated with stress and increase in adrenaline secretion.

Several other drugs are used to treat more difficult and serious heart rhythm disorders. Most of these drugs have serious side effects, are only 60 to 80 percent effective in controlling the disturbance, and they do not prevent death. Thus, doctors are not keen to treat extra beats unless they are associated with serious heart disease, especially coronary heart disease. In such patients, when extra beats are numerous with runs of three or more occurring together (ventricular tachycardia) drugs are usually tried.

Dosages of the drugs are not given here since they are a specialized group of drugs and cardiologists must control and individualize the dosage.

## Amiodarone

This is an experimental drug in the United States but has been used extensively in South America and Europe since 1974. The drug is very effective in suppressing life-threatening abnormal heart rhythms.

### Advice and Adverse Effects

The drug's major toxicity includes deposits of granules in the cornea, fibrosis of the lung in about 5 percent, and grayish blue discoloration of the skin with prolonged use at high doses.

Amiodarone must not be used in combination with verapamil. Interaction may occur when used concomitantly with quinidine, digoxin, and oral anticoagulants such as warfarin.

## Disopyramide

This drug has similar effects as quinidine. It is useful in the emergency treatment of ventricular tachycardia when given intravenously. Oral treatment suppresses extra beats in about 50 percent of cases.

### Advice and Adverse Effects

The drug should not be used in patients with heart failure or poor heart muscle function since it can precipitate heart failure. The drug is contraindicated in individuals with glaucoma, kidney failure, low blood pressure, and enlargement of the prostate because urinary retention can be precipitated. The drug must not be used in combination with verapamil.

## Lidocaine (lignocaine)

This drug is used intravenously in emergency situations and is very effective in suppressing ventricular tachycardia and serious extra beats. A relatively nontoxic drug, it is discussed in Chapter 10, "How to Deal with Heart Attacks."

## Mexiletine

This drug is more effective than disopyramide. It suppresses complex abnormal heart rhythm but it has not improved survival rate.

### Advice and Adverse Effects

Mexiletine is contraindicated in patients with low blood pressure. The dose must be reduced if kidney failure is present. Side effects include slowing of the pulse, stomach problems, confusional states, double vision, and disturbance in walking (ataxia). The drug is therefore reserved for the treatment of life-threatening arrythmias.

## Procainamide

Procainamide has similarities to the well-known quinidine. It is of value when given intravenously in the emergency management of ventricular tachycardia. That is not responsive to lidocaine. When used orally it has a variable effect. It is less effective than quinidine or disopyramide and when used for longer than six months, patients can develop joint pains and fever (lupus erythematosus). As well, although very rare, the white blood cells can be damaged (agranulocytosis). I rarely advise its oral use mainly because of its minimal effectiveness and side effects.

The drug should not be used in patients with low blood pressure, severe heart failure, and myastenia gravis.

## Quinidine

The use of quinidine has greatly decreased since 1975, especially since the advent of disopyramide and other anti-arrhythmic agents. However, it is one of the few agents that can be used safely, albeit cautiously, in patients with heart failure. In the Boston Collaborative Study, 652 patients taking quinidine had no exacerbation of heart failure despite a predrug incidence of 35 percent.[14] In the presence of heart failure, quinidine, mexiletine, and amiodarone are relatively safe drugs and do not depress the function of the heart muscle as do many other anti-arrhythmic agents.

The drug suppresses extra beats in about 60 percent of cases but is only partially effective with life-threatening arrhythmias. However, because the drug has been used for more than twenty-five years, it is still a commonly used drug for the treatment of abnormal rhythms.

### Advice and Adverse Effects

Quinidine can precipitate ventricular fibrillation, which is the most dangerous abnormal heart rhythm. It does not seem reasonable to give priority to a drug that may increase the risk of ventricular fibrillation and death. Quinidine may precipitate ventricular tachycardia and cardiac arrest.[15]

Quinidine increases the level of digoxin in the blood and when used concomitantly, care is necessary with digoxin and anticoagulants such as warfarin.

## *Tocainide*

This drug is similar to lidocaine, which is given intravenously. When given by mouth, tocainide is as effective as quinidine and possibly mexiletine.

Nausea, vomiting, constipation, and abdominal pain are common side effects; nervous system signs and rarely fibrosis of the lung may occur.


## CONCLUSION

We have a long way to go in the management of simple extra beats, more complex extra beats, ventricular tachycardia, and most importantly, the prevention of ventricular fibrillation, which is the cause of death in the majority of heart patients.

Questions still to be answered include the following:

1. Are the drugs effective in suppressing the abnormal rhythm?
2. Do they prevent ventricular fibrillation and prolong life, especially during and after a heart attack?
3. How serious are their side effects including the precipitation of more dangerous heart rhythms, even if the occurrence is rare?
4. Is their use justified in the given individual?

At present, partial success with the use of complex drug combinations in the seriously ill has been achieved, yet life has not been prolonged. In addition to toxicity, several visits to the doctor and cost must be justified. However, unless we continue to treat such seriously ill heart patients with the feeling that we can offer them some hope, we will never know when a new drug has the potential to save life. Therefore, it is noble that some patients persist with the use of experimental drug regimes to treat their life-threatening arrhythmias.

# CHAPTER 16

# DISEASES OF HEART VALVES

The valves of the heart are shown in Figure 1-2. The valves are like automatic doors, which open when people want to pass through and stay shut when not in use. When blood must be expelled from the left ventricle into the aorta, the aortic valve opens.

The valve texture is smooth so that blood particles and bacteria do not adhere to them. However, the valves may be the site of disease. When affected by disease, the soft valve tissue gets rough, thick, swollen, and hard, and as blood rushes through the obstructing or damaged valves, turbulence occurs. The turbulence sets up vibrations that are louder than normal and can be heard easily with the stethoscope. The sound heard by the stethoscope is called a murmur. The loudness of the murmur depends on the velocity of blood flow, the amount of blood passing across the deformed valve, and the turbulence that occurs.

## CAUSES OF VALVE DISEASE—MURMURS

Heart valve disease can be due to one of the following:

1. Rheumatic heart disease.
2. Infections, in particular, bacterial endocarditis and syphilis; fortunately, viral infection, though extremely common, is not known to cause valve disease.

3.   Rare congenital heart disease.
4.   Others: coronary heart disease, mitral valve prolapse, and degenerative diseases due to age changes, such as calcific aortic sclerosis.


Consequences of valve disease—*murmurs:*

1.   A murmur is produced and is easily heard by the doctor. Murmurs are most commonly systolic in time; that is, they occur during the contraction of the ventricles. Many systolic murmurs are not significant in that they do not disturb the function of the heart. However, murmurs that occur when the ventricles are relaxed, that is, during diastole, are termed diastolic murmurs and are always of significance.
2.   Over a period of five to fifty years, significant murmurs increase the work of the heart muscle and causes it to enlarge. The muscle finally becomes weak and heart failure occurs. When heart failure occurs, it is not the end of the life, as mentioned in Chapter 14.
3.   Infections may occur on the valve; this is called bacterial endocarditis.
4.   Complications due to obstruction or backward leak of blood may cause severe shortness of breath and surgery may be required in a few.
5.   Roughness of the valve may also extend into the chamber of the left atrium and set up discharges. Thus extra beats and palpitations including paroxysmal atrial tachycardia (PAT) and atrial fibrillation may occur.
6.   The major symptoms of serious valve disease are increasing shortness of breath, cough, and occasionally blood-tinged sputum (hemoptysis). Finally, signs of heart failure occur, and these include shortness of breath, edema of the legs, and water in and on the lungs.

## Diagnosis of Heart Murmur and Test Required

Usually the diagnosis is obvious from the patient's history of shortness of breath and the finding of a murmur with the stethoscope. A cardiologist makes the diagnosis in the office with 95 percent confidence in more than 95 percent of cases. The chest X-ray, ECG, and echocardiogram are helpful to confirm the opinion.

In a few individuals with serious heart murmurs causing symptoms such as severe shortness of breath with or without heart failure, catheter tests are invaluable and must be done if surgical correction is planned. The technique of catheterization is outlined in Chapter 11.

# RHEUMATIC HEART DISEASE

Damage to heart valves commonly occurs during an attack of rheumatic fever. Rheumatic fever is most common between the ages of five and twenty-five and occurs in susceptible individuals after a streptococcal sore throat. The streptococcus bacteria sets up an allergic-like reaction on the valves and in the joints. Fever, joint pains, and murmurs heard over the heart valves and a blood test to show a reaction to the streptococcus usually confirms the diagnosis.

Fortunately, sore throats caused by the streptococcus have become much less common and the disease is disappearing from North America. The disease persists in the Canadian far north and third-world countries. Not all individuals who get rheumatic fever develop damage to the heart valves. Those who have severe fever with marked involvement of the joints with severe joint pains lasting several months may never get valve damage. The opposite is most likely to occur: it appears that rheumatic fever when it "licks the joints spares the heart."

The mitral valve is commonly affected followed by the aortic valve. Other valves very rarely get damaged.

The valve lesions are the following:

## Mitral Stenosis

The silky, soft leaflets of the mitral valve become thickened, rough, and hard, and over a few years the orifice of the valve becomes tight. Blood in the left atrium has difficulty getting through the mitral valve to reach the left ventricle. When the orifice is severely narrowed, blood backs up into the lung and causes severe shortness of breath.

The treatment of mitral stenosis is surgery, which is necessary only if severe shortness of breath is present and persistent. Surgery is relatively simple and safe; the valve is opened with a finger or a special metal dilator. In a few cases the valve has to be removed and replaced by a prosthesis. The results of surgery are excellent but reserved for patients with severe symptoms. Many patients can live five to fifty years with mild to moderate symptoms before they become serious enough to warrant surgery. Severe complications are rare except when atrial fibrillation occurs; clots may then develop in the left atrium and these can move to the brain. When atrial fibrillation is not present, the prognosis is excellent.

## Mitral Regurgitation

The valve may be diseased in such a manner that it does not close tightly during contraction of the left ventricle. When the mitral valve is not shut tight, blood leaks or regurgitates from the ventricle back into the left atrium thus the leaking valve is called mitral regurgitation. These patients tolerate the leak for many years and, in a few, the left ventricle as well as the left atrium can become enlarged; shortness of breath occurs and surgery to replace the valve may be necessary. Patients can tolerate the lesions for five to seventy years depending on its degree.

## Aortic Stenosis

In aortic stenosis, the aortic valve is tight and obstructs the flow of blood from the left ventricle into the aorta; less blood reaches the head. Symptoms such as dizziness and fainting may occur. The left ventricle tries to overcome the obstruction by pumping more forcefully, and over years, the muscle enlarges and finally fails. A few cases may require surgery; severe shortness of breath, fainting spells, enlargement of the left ventricle, or heart failure are indications for surgery. The diseased valve is removed and an aortic valve prosthesis is usually inserted. This is extensive surgery and is done only when justifiable. Any patient over age forty-five may have concomitant coronary heart disease and may require valve replacement as well as coronary artery bypass graft. This combination surgery carries a high risk.

## Aortic Regurgitation

In this condition, the valve remains widely open when it should be tightly closed, therefore blood regurgitates or leaks from the aorta backward into the left ventricle. The left ventricle has more work to do and over several years dilates and enlarges. Surgery is not often required because the left ventricle copes with the extra work for many years. Leaking valves impose less work on the heart than obstructed valves. When heart failure occurs due to a leaking valve, digoxin and diuretics are helpful as well as vasodilators such as captopril and enalapril. Surgery is required in a few to replace the valve.

To reemphasize, a tight valve is medically called a stenosis, thus the terms "mitral stenosis" or "aortic stenosis." A leaky valve indicates regurgitation of blood, and the two common lesions are mitral regurgitation and aortic regurgitation. The pulmonary and tricuspid valve are very rarely affected except when due to congenital heart disease.

Prosthetic heart valve surgery is a major undertaking and careful assessment by a cardiology team is necessary. Post surgery, the patient may need to take anticoagulants to prevent clotting on the valve. Such clots can move to the brain or elsewhere in the body. Usually warfarin is given and some cardiologists add dipyridamole.

## CASE OF MRS. JB

At age twenty-nine this patient started having a cough with shortness of breath, mainly on climbing stairs. Over the next few weeks, symptoms occurred at night in bed. Cough, shortness of breath, and wheezing became worse over the next month, and her family doctor prescribed cough medicines. About one month later there was no improvement. At night she would have difficulty breathing and would have to sit up for a half to one hour to get some relief. The second visit to the doctor resulted in a twelve-day course of antibiotics and another cough medicine to clear the chest infection or congestion in the lungs.

I was treating her husband for hypertension, and he insisted that I see Mrs. B. I asked him to have the GP refer the patient. The patient's request was refused, and several weeks later she was no better; more cough medicine was prescribed along with an inhaler to try and relieve her bronchial spasms. There was no fever or chills. At this stage she had difficulty doing her housework and climbing stairs chiefly because of shortness of breath and cough. She noted that her sputum was tinged with blood at times. She smoked twenty to thirty cigarettes per day and was advised to give this up since she had bronchitis and congestion. I was requested again by the husband but since the system of practice is one by referral, I advised him to request the GP to get a consultation with a chest physician. The general practitioner refused to refer her to a chest physician and gave her another course of antibiotics and an inhaler.

At this stage, I saw the patient without a referral. Within less than a minute, the diagnosis was made in the office. There was no need to take further histories; a doctor who knows that the patient has shortness of breath usually listens to the chest (lungs) and the heart. She had the typical heart sounds and murmur of mitral stenosis. The valve was extremely tight, and blood was backing up, congesting and flooding the lungs. The general practitioner failed to distinguish congestion by blood, salt, and water, from that caused by infection. The chest X-ray was typical of mitral stenosis. I admitted her to the hospital that day. Her shortness of breath was 50 percent relieved by the diuretic furosemide and she was able to sleep. Her blood-tinged sputum disappeared over the next few days, and three weeks later she had heart catheterization. Cardiac surgery was performed the next month, the valve was opened, and five years later she remains healthy and able to do her housework and exercises. The lesson here is that a tight valve (mitral stenosis) and heart failure can mimic other causes of lung congestion and can produce symptoms that resemble asthma and acute bronchitis.

## Calcific Aortic Sclerosis

The aortic valve may become calcified and hardened (scle-rosed), especially during ages sixty to eighty, and the doctor may hear the loud murmur with a stethoscope. Fortunately the deposits of calcium do not cause significant obstruction to the blood flow. Thus this calcific valve very rarely becomes tight enough to cause symptoms, and tests are rarely required. Surgery may be necessary in 1 out of 10,000 cases. More than 33 percent of individuals over age seventy have a murmur over the aortic valve due to calcific aortic sclerosis. My grandmother had such a murmur and so did my dad; the murmurs sounded the same.

## Mitral Valve Prolapse

This is a common disease. The mitral valve leaflets become very soft and floppy. With a stethoscope, the doctor hears the valves flapping like a sail in a crisp wind. The noise heard is typical and is called a click and murmur. The click can be similar to a loud tick of a clock or at times it is a musical sound. The condition is somewhat more common in females, and about five percent of individuals over age twenty-five have this click and murmur, which is produced by the mitral valve and termed mitral valve prolapse.

The condition is very benign and only 1 in every 1,000 cases may have a problem. A few individuals may have palpitations consisting chiefly of extra beats (see Chapter 15). Chest pain is said to occur in a few but the condition is not related to coronary heart disease and there is no clear-cut relation between the disease and heart attacks. In less than 1 in 1,000 cases the valve leaflet may weaken or get a redundant fold and cause regurgitation of blood; in such patients mild mitral regurgitation may occur. Infection of the valve causing bacterial endocarditis and further damage may occur. Prophylaxis with antibiotics is advisable before dental work and surgical procedures; otherwise the patient, who can live to ninety, may have an abrupt shortening of life.

## BACTERIAL ENDOCARDITIS

Valves previously affected by rheumatic fever are thick, rough, and swollen. Other causes of deformity of the heart valves have been discussed. Bacteria that gain entry into the blood stream on their way through the heart may attach to the roughened valve surface and set up an area of infection. The bacteria may grow to form an "abcess" on the valve. The abcess resembles a clump of moss that swings and sways on the valve leaflet as it opens and closes. Pieces can dislodge and go to organs such as the brain or the kidneys. Infection of heart valves is called endocarditis. Usually the infection is by bacteria, therefore the term bacterial endocarditis.

In susceptible individuals, bacterial endocarditis can begin after simple manipulations such as scaling and cleaning of teeth, root canal, and other dental work. Patients who have mild heart valve lesions and can live a normal life to age ninety may get caught in the trap and their lives can be suddenly shortened by this infection.

### Case I

Mrs. S, age 69, had a fever of 100 to 104°F with chills and weakness over a period of fourteen months. She had attended several clinics and physicians including one period of hospitalization. She was previously quite well and was not known to have heart disease. She had six children; they were alive and healthy, and it was a surprise to them that their previously healthy mother was now bedridden. She was not short of breath and there was no cough. I was requested to see the patient. The diagnosis was obvious. The woman had a soft systolic murmur at the apex of the heart and typical swelling of the fingertips near the nail bed called finger clubbing. Clubbing is a hallmark of bacterial endocarditis. On questioning, she admitted that fourteen months previously she had had all her teeth removed. I treated her with a combination of penicillin and streptomycin for a period of six weeks and she made an uneventful recovery; ten years later she was alive and well.

Carious teeth and dental work can maim individuals with heart valve defects. Importantly, the heart valve defect may be a very mild one of very little significance causing no symptoms and yet can become infected. Individuals who have heart murmurs or valve clicks should receive antibiotic coverage to prevent endocarditis. This is discussed shortly.

## Case II

One unfortunate morning in 1973, LH, a twenty-nine-year-old female who was known to have a soft heart murmur, was walking to the bathroom and fell to the floor. Her left arm felt weak and her speech was slurred. She was rushed to the hospital, and after three days she had made a complete recovery and was discharged. Her father had had two heart attacks and was a patient of mine and he requested that I see her. The general practitioner refused referral, stating that it was a hysterical attack.

I saw the patient three weeks later at the insistence of her father. Like Mrs. S in case I, she had the typical features of finger clubbing, murmur, and fever. I admitted her to the hospital. She had a temperature of 100 to 102° F. Her blood was taken and cultured and grew a bacteria called streptococcus viridans; this is the most common cause of bacterial endocarditis. She was treated with penicillin and streptomycin for six weeks and made a good recovery. Her previous mild mitral valve regurgitation became moderate. Twelve years later, she is able to do her housework with mild exercises and enjoys life with some restrictions. She realizes that surgery will become necessary sometime in the next five years when she will have the valve replaced. However, you must note how long she has gone without a valve replacement.

## Case III

I.T., a forty-one-year-old female patient of mine since 1969, was known to have rheumatic fever at ages nine and seventeen. She had had a moderate degree of mitral regurgitation since 1966. In 1983 at age thirty-nine she wanted to have a baby. Because of the risk of pregnancy at her age and a serious murmur, a heart catheter test was done that showed moderate to severe mitral regurgitation. She insisted on the pregnancy and, surprisingly, did extremely well. About two years later during an unfortunate month of May 1985, she had a fever of 100 to 102°F with chills. She had a lack of energy and visited her general practitioner. After a couple of visits to her doctor, her spleen was found to be slightly enlarged. Because of the spleen and mild anemia, she was referred to a blood specialist (hematologist). However, a few days before the appointment, while at work, she had moderate to severe chest pain and summoned my assistance. I rushed her to the emergency room and had her admitted. She had a temperature of 102 to 104°F; she looked ill, and she had the typical features of bacterial endocarditis, that is, fever, a murmur, and mild finger clubbing. The spleen gets slightly enlarged and low blood count (anemia) may occur in more than 60 percent of patients with endocarditis.

Her blood was cultured and grew streptococcus viridans. She was started on intravenous antibiotics. Echocardiography showed vegetations on the mitral valve, and one of the vegetations seemed to float back and forth. I recommended an immediate valve replacement. A prosthetic heart valve was inserted. Two months follow-up in the office revealed a normal functioning prosthetic heart valve and a pleasant, satisfied patient.

I must emphasize that apart from infection of previously damaged heart valves as well as prosthetic valves, normal valves can become damaged. Fortunately this occurs extremely rarely and mainly in drug addicts. The syringe and needles may be contaminated, and germs introduced into the bloodstream can infect valves on the right side of the heart (tricuspid and pulmonary valves). These germs are very actively growing types; thus, they can damage normal valves. The bacteria found in such cases are staphylococcus and pseudomonas.

## PREVENTION OF RHEUMATIC FEVER

Rheumatic fever tends to recur in the same individual. In order to prevent recurrence, the following is advised: If rheumatic fever was properly documented, but there is no evidence of valve damage, penicillin is usually given for a minimum of five years or to age twenty, whichever is longest. If the heart valve was damaged, penicillin is given for a minimum of ten years or to age forty, whichever is the longest. Depending on the state or country, and the prevalence of beta-hemolytic streptococci and rheumatic fever, some physicians continue treatment beyond age forty. The dose of antibiotic is usually one of the following:

1. Penicillin-V, 250 mg twice daily. If the patient is allergic to penicillin, sulfadiazine is as effective—1 g once daily for adults and 0.5 g daily for patients weighing less than sixty pounds.
2. 1.2 million units of benzathine penicillin G intramuscularly, given monthly.

## PREVENTION OF BACTERIAL ENDOCARDITIS

The American Heart Association recommendations for preventing bacterial endocarditis are as follows:

Patients with valvular heart disease must be given antibiotics a half to one hour prior to all dental or surgical procedures. The antibiotic is given orally for dental work done under local anesthetic. The antibiotic is given intramuscularly or intravenously for patients with prosthetic valves, patients with highest risk of developing endocarditis, or patients who are having a general anesthetic. All dental procedures that are likely to result in gingival bleeding such as extractions, root canal, scaling and cleaning, and surgery in the oral cavity require antibiotic coverage to prevent endocarditis.[16]

Oral therapy is given when a local anesthetic is used in patients not at high risk. The adult dose is 2 g of penicillin-V, taken orally an hour prior to the procedure, then 1 g six hours later.[16] Patients allergic to penicillin usually receive erythromycin or vancomycin.

For surgery on the intestine or the genital or urinary systems, other antibiotics are required intravenously. You must warn the doctor in the hospital that you have a murmur.

A British Society Working Party recommendation for endocarditis prevention during dental procedures recommends the following: When dental work is done under local anesthetic, if there is no allergy to penicillin, 3 gm of amoxycillin are taken orally in the presence of a dentist (1.5 g to children) one hour before the operation. If the surgery is done under general anesthetic for dental work and the patient is not allergic to penicillin, 1 g of amoxycillin is given intramuscularly or intravenously followed by 0.5 g orally six hours later.[17]

## Questions Posed

A female, age 30, posed the following questions: My family doctor says that I have a systolic murmur at the apex of the heart and referred me to a cardiologist. I would like to know:

1. What is my prognosis?
2. Is there any contraindication to using the birth control pill?
3. Will the murmur affect future pregnancy and the number of children I can have?
4. When will an operation be necessary?
5. Can I prevent it from becoming worse?

Answers

1. A soft systolic murmur over the apex of the heart is usually of no significance. It is important, however, to identify any mild area of roughness or deformity of the valve, which can later develop an infection called endocarditis. When a doctor states that a murmur is of no significance, it means that the murmur will not affect the person's lifespan or activities. If you have not had rheumatic fever and there are no other murmurs and no shortness of breath, the murmur is likely due to an increased blood flow across the valve, a common finding in young adults and also during pregnancy. The cardiologist's findings with the stethoscope, followed by a chest X-ray and electrocardiogram usually exclude most serious problems. If some doubt exists, an echocardiogram is helpful. Echocardiography will document a degree of stenosis, and if the machine is equipped with Doppler equipment, the degree of regurgitation can be documented. I must add that diastolic murmurs are always significant whereas soft systolic murmurs are usually not of significance.

2. The murmur does not contraindicate the use of the birth control pill. However, women over age thirty who smoke and take the birth control pill greatly increase their risk of developing blood clots.

3. The murmur will not affect your pregnancy, the fetus, or subsequent pregnancies and should not limit the number of children. If the murmur is loud and the doctor hears it over a wide area around the apex and around the axilla and near the left shoulder blade, this is a different matter and further assessment is necessary to exclude significant mitral regurgitation.

4. An operation is nearly never required in patients with a soft systolic murmur or mild mitral regurgitation. Surgery for mitral regurgitation is utilized only when there are symptoms of severe shortness of breath or heart enlargement and when a Doppler echo shows severe regurgitation that is confirmed by catheter test.

5. If you have no symptoms and if the murmur is described as soft and heard over an area of less than five

or ten fingertips held together, it is most unlikely that your condition will get worse. Only infection of the valve can shorten your life. Fortunately, the risk of getting an infection on the valve is remote; when germs get into the blood, they need to stick on the valve and grow. However, there is a 1 in 1,000 chance of this occurring, and prevention through antibiotics is the rule. (See recommendations at the beginning of this section.)

*Preventive medicine* has helped to irradicate the dreadful streptococcus not only by the use of antibiotics but through the relief of overcrowding and the improvement of sanitation in disadvantaged socioeconomic groups. Thus, rheumatic fever is now rare in North America. Similarly, we can prevent bacterial endocarditis by intelligent use of appropriate antibiotics on the day of dental or other surgery. The rare, very serious valve disorder can be cured surgically in the majority of cases. Heart valve disease is becoming uncommon, and valve surgery has certainly progressed in the past twenty years. We cannot say the same for the prevention of coronary heart disease, but our fight must continue, especially if we commence preventive measures in childhood.

# CONCLUSIONS

The artificial heart of year 2086 will not be equivalent or superior to the healthy human heart. A successful artificial heart available in that year will likely be capable of saving, at most, 5,000 lives around the world. Visualize 5,000 surgical operations to implant the fantastic device. Compare 6 million deaths per year from heart attacks. Three million occur within one hour, that is, before medical help is available. These deaths are due to blockage of a coronary artery by a combination of atherosclerosis and blood clots.

Thus, we must invest huge amounts of money and engage in more research to find the exact causes of atherosclerosis and coronary thrombosis to deal effectively with their prevention.

Public education will need to be continuous and current if prevention is to succeed.

*Protect the hearts of your children.* Start at least from age ten in schools and in the home to educate children about the magnitude of the problem and its prevention. The epidemic is as dangerous as a nuclear war. Consider that over the next 100 years there will be 600 million deaths from heart attacks if we do not halt the epidemic.

We are faced with a major task of educating the public from childhood about protection of the heart, if we are to curb the epidemic of heart disease.

I hope that I have given you some insight and suitable practical advice and methods to help prevent a heart attack. As well, your reading of this book should increase your knowledge of the treatment of heart disease and high blood pressure, and this should assist you along with the help of your doctor.

This is not a pill book that lists numerous drugs, their side effects, and manufacturers' proclamations. I have given you, as it were, a consumer report. The relative merits of various drugs are discussed. Comparisons are made so that in consultation with your doctor you can assess whether or not the particular drug is useful and its use justified, or whether the drugs' use is not justifiable.

# REFERENCES

## PART I

1. The Norwegian Multicenter Study Group: Timolol-induced reduction in mortality and reinfarction in patients surviving acute myocardial infarction. N Engl J Med 304:801, 1981.
2. DeWood MA, Spores J, Notske R, et al: Prevalence of total coronary occlusion during the early hours of transmural myocardial infarction. N Engl J Med 303:897, 1980.
3. Davies MJ, Thomas A: Thrombosis and acute coronary-artery lesions in sudden cardiac ischemic death. N Engl J Med 310:1137, 1984.
4. Duguid JB: Cholesterol. Br J Hosp Med 286, 1980.
5. The Lipid Research Clinics Program: The Lipid Research Clinics Coronary Primary Prevention Trial Results: I. The relationship of reduction in incidence of coronary heart disease to cholesterol lowering. JAMA 251:365, 1984.
6. Rose G: Strategy of prevention: lessons from cardiovascular disease. Br Med J 282: 1847, 1981.
7. Keyes A: Seven Countries—A Multivariate Analysis of Death and Coronary Heart Disease. Cambridge, Mass., Harvard University Press, 1980.
8. Kannel WB, Castelli WP, Gordon T: Cholesterol in the prediction of atherosclerotic disease. New perspectives based on the Framingham Study. Ann Intern Med 90:85, 1979a.
9. Brensike JF, Levy RI, Kelsey SF, et al.: Effects of therapy with cholestyramine on progression of coronary arteriosclerosis: results of the NHLBI Type II Coronary Intervention Study. Circulation 69:313, 1984.

311

10. Durrington PN: High-density lipoprotein cholesterol: methods and clinical significance. CRC Crit Rev in Clin Lab Sci 18:31, 1983.

11. Harris WS, Connor WE, McMurry MP: The comparative reduction of the plasma lipids and lipoproteins by dietary polyunsaturated fats: salmon oil versus vegetable oil. Metabolism 32:179, 1983.

12. Hirai A, Hamazaki T, Terano T, et al.: Eicosapentaenoic acid and platelet function in Japanese. Lancet II:1132, 1980.

13. Siess W, Roth P, Scherer B, et al.: Platelet-membrane fatty acids, platelet aggregation, and thromboxane formation during a mackerel diet. Lancet I:441, 1980.

14. Menon IS, Kendal RY, Dewar HA, et al.: Effect of onions on blood fibrinolytic activity. Br Med J 5614:351, 1968.

15. Trustwell AS: End of a static decade for coronary disease? Br Med J 289:509, 1984.

16. The basics of the prudent diet: Heartbook, The American Heart Association. New York, E. P. Dutton, 1980.

17. Coronary Drug Project Research Group: Coronary Drug Project: clofibrate and niacin in coronary heart disease. JAMA 231:360, 1975.

18. Coronary Drug Project Research Group: Coronary Drug Project: findings leading to further modifications of its protocol with respect to dextrothyroxine. JAMA 220:996, 1972.

19. Castelli WP, Garrison RJ, Dawber TR, et al., The filter cigarette and coronary heart disease: The Framingham Study. Lancet II: 109, 1981.

20. Wald NJ, Idle M, Boreham J, et al.: Serum cotinine levels in pipe smokers: evidence against nicotine as cause of coronary heart disease. Lancet II:775, 1981.

21. Multiple Risk Factor Intervention Trial Research Group: Multiple risk factor intervention trial: risk factor changes and mortality results. JAMA 248:1465, 1982.

22. Feinleib M, Williams RR: Relative risks of myocardial infarction, cardiovascular disease and peripheral vascular disease by type of smoking. Proc. Third World Conf. Smoking and Health I: 243, 1976.

23. Cryer PE, Haymond MW, Santiago JV, et al.: Norepinephrine and epinephrine release and adrenergic medication of smoking—associated hemodynamic and metabolic events. N Engl J Med 295:573, 1986.

24. Wald NJ, Howard S, Smith PG, et al.: Association between atherosclerotic distress and carboxyhemoglobin levels in tobacco smokers. Br Med J I:761, 1973.

25.   Kannell WB: Cigarettes, coronary occlusions and myocardial infarction. JAMA 246:871, 1981a.

26.   DeBias DA, Banerjee CM, Birkhead NC, et al.: Effects of carbon monoxide inhalation on ventricular fibrillation. Arch Environ Health 31:38, 1976.

27.   Aronow WS, Stemmer EA, Zweig S: Carbon monoxide and ventricular fibrillation threshold in normal dogs. Arch Environ Health 34:184, 1979.

28.   Aronow WS: Effect of non-nicotine cigarettes and carbon monoxide on angina. Circulation 61:262, 1980.

29.   Russell MAH, Raw M. Jarvis MJ: Clinical use of nicotine chewing-gum. Br Med J 1:1599–1602, 1980.

30.   Virag R, Bouilly P, Frydman D: Is impotence an arterial disorder. Lancet I:181, 1985.

31.   Hurd PD, Johnson CA, Pechacek T, et al.: Prevention of cigarette smoking in seventh grade students. J Behav Med 3:15, 1980.

32.   Paffenbarger RS Jr, Hale WE: Work activity and coronary heart mortality. N Engl J Med 292:545, 1975.

33.   Morris JN, Hagan A, Patterson DC, et al.: Incidence and prediction of ischemic heart disease in London busmen. Lancet II:553, 1966.

34.   Paffenbarger RS Jr, Wing AL, Hyde RT; Physical activity as an index of heart attack risk in college allumni. Am J Epidemiol 108:161, 1978.

35.   Sedgwick AN, Brotherhood JR, Davidson A, et al.: Long-term effects of physical training programme on risk factors for coronary heart disease in otherwise sedentary men. Br Med J 281:7, 1980.

36.   Morris JN, Everitt MG, Pollard R, et al.: Vigorous exercise in leisure-time: protection against coronary heart disease. Lancet I:1207, 1980.

37.   Milvey P, Siegel AJ: Physical activity levels and altered mortality from coronary heart disease with an emphasis on marathon running: A critical review. Cardiovasc Rev 2:233, 1981.

38.   Siscovick DS, Weiss NS, Fletcher RH, et al.: The incidence of primary cardiac arrest during vigorous exercise. N Engl J Med 311:874, 1984.

39.   Thompson PD, Funk EJ, Carleton RA, et al.: Incidence of death during jogging in Rhode Island from 1975 through 1980. JAMA 247:2535, 1982.

40.   Waller BF, Roberts WC: Sudden death while running in conditioned runners aged 40 years or over. Am J Cardiol 45:1292, 1980.

41.  Thompson PD, Stern WP, Williams P, et al.: Death during jogging or running: study of 18 cases. JAMA 242:1265, 1979.

42.  Haskell WL: Physical activity and health: need to define the required stimulus. AM J Cardiol 55:4D, 1985.

43.  Selye H: Stress Without Distress. Philadelphia, J. B. Lippincott, 1974.

44.  Deanfield JE, Shea M, Kensett M, et al.: Silent myocardial ischemia due to mental stress. Lancet II:1001, 1984.

45.  Sinatra ST, Feitell LA: The heart and mental stress, real and imagined. Lancet I:222, 1985.

46.  Haft JI, Fani K: Intravascular platelet aggregation in the heart induced by stress. Circulation 47:353, 1973.

47.  Haft JI, Fani K: Stress and the induction of intravascular platelet aggregation in the heart. Circulation 48:164, 1973.

48.  Satinsky J, Kowsowsky B, Lown B: Ventricular fibrillation induced by hypothalmic stimulation during coronary occlusion. Circulation Supplement II, 11, 1971.

49.  Khan, MI, Hamilton JT, Manning GW: Protective effect of beta adrenoceptor blockade in experimental coronary occlusion in conscious dogs. Am J Cardiol 30:832, 1972.

50.  Lown B, De Silva RA, Reech P, et al.: Psychophysiologic factors in sudden cardiac death. Am J Psych 137, 1325, 1980.

51.  Keys A: Overweight, Obesity, Coronary Heart Disease and Mortality, Nutrition Reviews 38:297, 1980.

52.  Kannel WB, Gordon T: Physiological and medical concomitants of obesity; the Framingham Study. In Bray GA (ed): Obesity in America. DHEW Publication No (NIH) 79, Washington, DC, US Government Printing Office, 1979.

53.  Bray GA: Obesity in America. DHEW Publications No (NIH) 79–359. Washington, DC, US Government Printing Office, 1979b.

54.  Eyton A: The F-Plan Diet. New York, Bantam Books, 1984.

55.  Eastwood MA, Passmore R: Dietary fibre. Lancet II:202, 1983.

56.  Stunkard AJ, Craighead LW, O'Brien R: Controlled trial of behavioral therapy, pharmacotherapy and their combination in the treatment of obesity. Lancet II:1045, 1980.

57.  Isner JM, Sours HE, Pares AL, et al.: Sudden, unexpected death in avid dieters using the liquid-protein–modified-fast diet. Circulation 60:1401, 1979.

58.  The very low calorie diet. Lancet II:500, 1984.

59.  Gordon TG, Kannel WB, Hjortland MC, et al.: Menopause and coronary heart disease: The Framingham Study. Ann Intern Med 89:157, 1978.

60. Coronary Drug Project Research Group: The Coronary Drug Project. Findings leading to discontinuation of the 2.5 mg/day estrogen group. JAMA 226, 652, 1973.

61. Ross RK, Mack TM, Paganini-Hill A, et al.: Menopausal estrogen therapy and protection from death and ischaemic heart disease. Lancet I:858, 1981.

62. Shapiro S, Slone D, Rosenberg L, et al.: Oral-contraceptive use in relation to myocardial infarction. Lancet I:743, 1979.

63. Friedman M, Rosenman RH: Type A Behavior and Your Heart. New York, Alfred A. Knopf, 1974.

64. Rosenman RH, Brand RT, Sholtz RI, et al.: Multivariate prediction of coronary heart disease during 8.5 year follow-up in the Western Collaborative Group Study. Am J Cardiol 37:903, 1976.

65. Review Panel on Coronary-Prone Behavior and Coronary Heart Disease. Coronary-prone behavior and coronary heart disease. A critical review. Circulation 63:1199, 1981.

66. Case RB, Heller SS, Case NB, et al.: Type A behavior and survival after acute myocardial infarction. N Engl J Med 312: 737, 1985.

67. Keatingé WR, Coleshaw SRK, Cotter F, et al.: Increase in platelet and red cell counts, blood viscosity, and arterial pressure during mild surface cooling: factors in mortality from coronary and cerebral thrombosis in winter. Br Med J 289:1405, 1984.

68. Meade TW: Review of the present status of antithrombotic drug therapy. In Coltart J, Jewitt DE (eds): Recent Developments in Cardiovascular Drugs, p. 259. Edinburgh, Churchill Livingstone, 1982.

69. Lewis HD, Davis JW, Archibald DG, et al: Protective effects of aspirin against acute myocardial infarction and death in men with unstable angina: results of a Veterans Administration Cooperative Study. N Engl J Med 309:396, 1983.

70. Anturane Reinfarction Trial Research Group: Sulfinpyrazone in the prevention of cardiac death after myocardial infarction: The Anturane Reinfarction Trial. N Engl J Med 298:289, 1978.

71. Furberg CD, Friedewald WT, Eberlein KA (eds): Proceedings of the Workshop on Implications of Recent Beta-Blockers Trials for Post-Myocardial Infarction Patients. Circulation Part II, 67, 1983.

72. Khan MG: Manual of Cardiac Drug Therapy, p. 119. London, Baillière Tindall, 1984.

# PART II

1. Pantridge JF, Geddes JS: Diseases of the cardiovascular system. Management of acute myocardial infarction. Br Med J 2:168, 1976.

2. Cobb LA, Baum RS, Alvarez H, et al.: Resuscitation from out of hospital ventricular fibrillation: 4 years follow-up. Circulation Supplement II, 51–52:223, 1975.

3. Van de Werf F, Ludbrook PA, Bergmann SR, et al.: Coronary thrombolysis with tissue-type plasminogen activator in patients with evolving myocardial infarction. N Engl J Med 310:610, 1984.

4. The TIMI Study Group: The thrombolysis in myocardial infarction (TIMI) trial. N Engl J Med 312:932, 1985.

5. The Norwegian Multicenter Study Group: Timolol-induced reduction in mortality and reinfarction in patients surviving acute myocardial infarction. N Engl J Med 304:801, 1981.

6. Furberg CD, Friedewald WT, Eberlein KA (eds): Proceedings of the Workshop on Implications of Recent Beta-Blocker Trials for Post-Myocardial Infarction Patients. Circulation Part II, 67: 1983.

7. Baber NS, Julian DG, Lewis JA, et al.: Beta-blockers after myocardial infarction: have trials changed practice? Br Med J 289:1431, 1984.

8. Thadani U, Fung HL, Darke AC, et al.: Oral isosorbide dinitrate in angina pectoris: comparison of duration of action and dose-response relation during acute and sustained therapy. Am J Cardiol 49:411, 1982.

9. Khan MG: Management of angina pectoris. In Manual of Cardiac Drug Therapy, p. 78. London, Baillière Tindall, 1984.

10. Carr AA, Mulligan OF, Sherrill LN: Pindolol versus methyldopa for hypertension: comparison of adverse reactions. Am Heart J 104:479, 1982.

11. Fleckenstein A: Specific pharmacology of calcium in myocardium, cardiac pacemakers, and vascular smooth muscle. Annu Rev Pharmacol Toxicol 17:149, 1977.

12. Campeau L, Enjarbest M, Lesperance J, et al.: The relation of risk factors to the development of atherosclerosis in saphenous-vein bypass grafts and the progression of disease in the native circulation. A study 10 years after aorto-coronary bypass surgery. N Engl J Med 311:1329, 1984.

13. William VL: Percutaneous transluminal coronary angioplasty, a 1985 perspective. Circulation 71:189, 1985.

14. The expanding scope of coronary angioplasty. Lancet I:1307, 1985.
15. American Heart Association: Standards and guidelines for cardio-pulmonary resuscitation (CPR) and emergency cardiac care (ECC). JAMA 244:453, 1980.
16. Khan MG: Cardiac Arrest. In Manual of Cardiac Drug Therapy, p. 191. London, Baillière Tindall, 1984.

# PART III

1. deWardener HE: Salt and hypertension. Lancet II:688, 1984.
2. Brown JJ, Lever AF, Robertson TIS, et al.: Salt and hypertension. Lancet II:456, 1984.
3. Hypertension Detection and Follow-up Program Cooperative Group: Five-year findings of the hypertension detection and follow-up program: I. Reduction in mortality of persons with high blood pressure, including mild hypertension. JAMA 242:2562, 1979.
4. The Australian Therapeutic Trial in Mild Hypertension: Report by the Management Committee. Lancet I:1261, 1980.
5. Multiple Risk Factor Intervention Trial Research Group: Multiple risk factor intervention trial: risk factor changes and mortality results. JAMA 248:1465, 1982.
6. Spence JD: Effects of antihypertensive agents on blood velocity: implications for atherogenesis. Can Med Assoc J 127:721, 1982.
7. Norwegian Multicenter Study Group: Timolol-induced reduction in mortality and reinfarction in patients surviving acute myocardial infarction, N Engl J Med 304:801, 1981.
8. Khan MG: Management of hypertension. In Manual of Cardiac Drug Therapy, p. 55. London, Ballière Tindall, 1984.
9. Murphy MB, Lewis PJ, Kohner E, et al.: Glucose intolerance in hypertensive patients treated with diuretics: a fourteen-year follow-up. Lancet II:1293, 1982.
10. Veteran's Administration Cooperative Study Group on Antihypertensive Agents: Comparison of propranolol and hydrochlorothiazide for the initial treatment of hypertension: I. Results of short-term titration with emphasis on racial differences in response. JAMA 248:1996, 1982.
11. Floras JS, Jones JV, Hassan MO, Sleight P: Ambulatory blood pressure during once-daily randomised double-blind administra-

tion of atenolol, metoprolol, pindolol, and slow-release propranolol. Br Med J 285:1387, 1982.

12. Carr AA, Mulligan OF, Sherrill LN: Pindolol versus methyldopa for hypertension: comparison of adverse reactions. Am Heart J 104:479, 1982.

13. Baim DS, McDowell AV, Cherniles J, et al.: Evaluation of a new bipyridine inotropic agent—Milrinone—in patients with severe congestive heart failure. N Engl J Med 309:748, 1983.

14. Cohen IS, Jick H, Cohen SI: Adverse reactions to quinidine in hospitalized patients: findings based on data from the Boston Collaborative Drug Surveillance Program. Prog Cardiovasc Dis 20:151, 1977.

15. Ruskin JN, McGovern B, Garan H, et al.: Antiarrhythmic drugs: a possible cause of out-of-hospital cardiac arrest. N Engl J Med 309:1302, 1983.

16. Prevention of bacterial endocarditis: a statement for health professionals by the committee on rheumatic fever and infective endocarditis of the council on cardiovascular disease in the young. Circulation 70:1123A, 1984.

17. Simmons NA, Cawson RA, Clarke C, et al.: The antibiotic prophylaxis of inefective endocarditis. Report of a working party of the British Society for Antimicrobial Chemotherapy. Lancet II:1323, 1982.

# GLOSSARY

**Aneurysm:** A severe weakening of the wall of an artery or heart muscle, leading to a ballooning of the wall of the vessel or heart.

**Angina pectoris:** Chest pain due to severe but temporary lack of blood and oxygen to a part of the heart muscle.

**Aorta:** Main artery arising from the heart; the branches of the aorta take blood to all parts of the body.

**Arrhythmia:** General term for an irregularity or rapidity of the heartbeat.

**Arteriosclerosis:** Loss of elasticity and hardening of arteries due to all causes such as age change, deposits of calcium, or by deposits of atheroma.

**Artery:** Blood vessels that carry blood away from the heart to organs, tissues, and cells throughout the body, as opposed to *veins*, which carry blood from the tissues back to the heart.

**Atheroma:** A hardened plaque in the wall of an artery: the plaque is filled with cholesterol, calcium, and other substances. The plaque of atheroma hardens the artery, hence the term "atherosclerosis" (sclerosis-hardening).

**Atrium:** One of two upper chambers of the heart.

**Calorie:** A unit of energy; one calorie represents the amount of heat required to raise the temperature of one kilogram of water, one degree Celsius. The energy present in foods is measured in calories.

**Cardiac arrest:** Cessation of the heartbeat.

**Cardiac catheterization:** A cardiac catheter is inserted through a vein or artery and pushed and propelled to reach inside the heart. The progress of the catheter is watched on a fluoroscope.

**Catheter:** A flexible tube that can be inserted into body organs to achieve drainage, treatment, or diagnosis.

**Cholesterol:** A lipid, or fatlike substance, made by animal cells.

**Coronary thrombosis:** A blood clot in a coronary artery, blocking blood flow to a part of the heart muscle. Also called a heart attack or myocardial infarction.

**Embolism, embolus:** A blood clot or clump of platelets that forms in an artery, in a vein, or inside the heart and breaks off and is carried by the circulating blood, finally lodging and blocking the artery that supplies an organ with blood. For example, a pulmonary embolism is an embolus blocking an artery in the lung.

**Hemoglobin:** *Heme*—"iron," *globin*—"protein"; an iron-protein substance present in red blood cells that carries oxygen to the cells of the body.

**Infarct or infarction:** An area of cells that die as a result of blockage of an artery that brings blood to these cells.

**Ischemia:** Temporary lack of blood and oxygen to an area of cells (e.g., heart muscle) usually due to severe obstruction of the artery supplying blood to this area of cells. Thus the term "ischemic heart disease" is synonymous with coronary artery disease or coronary heart disease.

**Myocardial infarction (infarct):** Death of an area of heart muscle due to blockage of a coronary artery by blood clot and atheroma; medical term for a heart attack.

**Myocardium:** The heart muscle.

**Murmur:** A noise or extra sound heard between normal heartbeats. The doctor hears the sound with a stethoscope.

**Pericarditis:** Inflammation of the pericardium or sac surrounding the heart; this is not a heart attack.

**Pericardium:** The thin, tough membrane or sac that surrounds the heart.

**Platelets:** Very small disc-like particles that circulate in the blood and initiate the formation of blood clots. Platelets clump and form little plugs, thus stopping bleeding.

**Stroke:** Damage of part of the brain due to blockage or rupture of an artery in the brain, which leads to weakness or paralysis of limbs with or without disturbances of speech or consciousness. A stroke or cerebrovascular accident is not a form of heart attack.

**Ventricle:** One of the two lower chambers of the heart.

**Ventricular fibrillation:** The heart muscle does not contract but "quivers"; therefore, there is no heartbeat (cardiac arrest). No blood is pumped out of the heart. Death occurs within minutes if the abnormal heart rhythm is not corrected. Note that in atrial fibrillation, the atrium fibrillates but the ventricles contract normally although faster than normal; this condition is usually not life-threatening and is easily controlled with the commonly known heart drug, digoxin.

| GENERIC | PHARMACEUTICAL TRADE NAME |
|---|---|

Blood Pressure Pills
### Beta-Blockers (pages 243–247)

| | |
|---|---|
| Atenolol | Tenormin |
| Labetalol | Normodyne Trandate |
| Metoprolol | Betaloc, Lopressor |
| Nadolol | Corgard |
| Oxprenolol | Trasicor |
| Pindolol | Visken |
| Propranolol | Inderal, Inderal LA |
| Timolol | Blocadren, Betim |

### Diuretics (pages 247–249)

| | |
|---|---|
| Thiazides | Diuril, Saluric |
| Chlorothiazide | Hydrodiuril, Esidrix |
| Hydrochlorothiazide | Oretic, Direma |
| Bendrofluazide | Aprinox, Berkozide Centyl, Neo-Naclex |
| Chlorthalidone | Hygroton |
| Indapamide | Lozol, Natrilix |
| Metolazone | Xaroxolyn, Metenix |
| Strong diuretics | |
| Furosemide, frusemide | Lasix, Dryptal |
| Bumetanide | Burinex, Bumex |
| Ethacrynic acid | Edecrin |
| Diuretics that retain potassium | |
| Amiloride | Midamor |
| Spironolactone | Aldactone |
| Triamterene | Dyrenium Dytac |
| Thiazide combined with potassium-retaining diuretic | |
| Nongeneric names | Aldactazide Dyazide Moduretic, Moduret |

### Vasodilators (dilate arteries) (pages 249–255)

| | |
|---|---|
| Captopril | Capoten |
| Enalapril | Vasoril |
| Hydralazine | Apresoline |
| Nifedipine | Adalat, Procardia |
| Prazosin | Minipress, Hypovase |

Other antihypertensives

| | |
|---|---|
| Clonidine | Catapres |
| Guanabenz | Wytensin |
| Methyldopa | Aldomet, Dopamet, Hydromet, Medomet |
| Reserpine | Abicol, Decaserpyl, Endruronyl, Harmonyl, Raudixin, Rautrax, Serpasil, others |

## Drugs Used for Angina (pages 169–189)
Beta-Blockers
See above list.

## Calcium Antagonists (pages 182–189)

| | |
|---|---|
| Diltiazem | Anginyl, Cardizem, Dilzem |
| Nifedipine | Adalat, Procardia |
| Verapamil | Calan, Cordilox, Isoptin, Isoptino, Manidon, Vasolan |

## Nitrates (pages 169–174)

| | |
|---|---|
| Nitroglycerin (sublingual) | Nitrostat, Nitro-Bid, others |
| Isosorbid dinitrate | Coronex, Isordil, Sorbitrate, others |

## Drugs for Heart Failure (pages 270–275)

| | |
|---|---|
| Digoxin | Lanoxin, others |
| Furosemide and other diuretics | See above. |
| Vasodilators such as Captopril and Enalapril | |

## Drugs for Abnormal Heart Rhythms (Arrhythmias) (pages 290–294)

| | |
|---|---|
| Amiodarone | Cordarone, Cordarone X |
| Beta-blockers. See above. | |
| Digoxin | Lanoxin |
| Disopyramide | Norpace, Rythmodan |
| Mexiletine | Mexitil |
| Tocainide | Tonocard |
| Quinidine | Cardioquin, Quinidex, Quinate, Biquin Durules others |

## Drugs That Affect Blood Clotting (pages 90–93)
Blood thinners: Anticoagulants

| | |
|---|---|
| Warfarin | Coumadin, Warfilone, Marevan, others |

Reduce Stickiness of Blood Platelets (Not blood thinners)

| | |
|---|---|
| Acetylsalicylic acid | Aspirin; coated aspirin, Entrophen, Novasen |
| Dipyridamole | Persantin, Persantine, Cardoxin |
| Sulfinpyrazone | Anturan Anturane |
| Potassium supplements (See Table 14-2) | |

Drugs That Reduce Cholesterol or Triglycerides (pages 31–35)

| | |
|---|---|
| Cholestyramine | Questran, Cuemid, Quantalan |
| Colestipol | Colestid |
| Clofibrate | Atromid-S |
| Gemfibrozil | Lopid |
| Probucol | Lorelco, Lurselle Lesterol |

# APPENDIX B

## NORMAL VALUES OR NORMAL RANGE OF SOME BLOOD CONSTITUENTS

dl = deciliter = 100 ml of blood
mEq/L = milliequivalent per liter of blood
mmol/L = micromole per liter of blood

| | United States | | Canada (metric) |
|---|---|---|---|
| Cholesterol | 150 to 220 mg/dL | $\div$ 38.7 = | 3.7 to 5.7 mmol/L |
| HDL cholesterol | 40 to 80 mg/dL | $\div$ 38.7 = | 1 to 2 mmol/L |
| Creatinine | Less than 1.4 mg/dL | | Less than 130 $\mu$mol/l |
| (Test of kidney function) | | | |
| Potassium | 4 to 5 mEq/L | | 4 to 5 mmol/L |
| Triglycerides | 50 to 250 mg/dL | $\div$ 100 = | 0.5 to 2.5 mmol/L |

# INDEX

## ABOUT THE AUTHOR

M. Gabriel Khan is an associate Professor of Medicine, University of Ottawa and a consultant cardiologist with a practice in Ottawa since 1969. He obtained his medical degrees at: The Queen's University of Belfast in 1961 with first class honours, the membership of the Royal College of Physicians of London in 1963, a Doctorate in Medicine with honours in 1964 and Fellowship of the Royal College of Physicians of Canada in 1969. He has devoted many years caring for patients with heart and hypertensive disease. He firmly believes in prevention first and strives for a more intelligent use of drugs. Dr. Khan is a Fellow of the American College of Physicians and the author of a medical textbook, *Cardiac Drug Therapy*, which has attained world-wide distribution and acclaim.